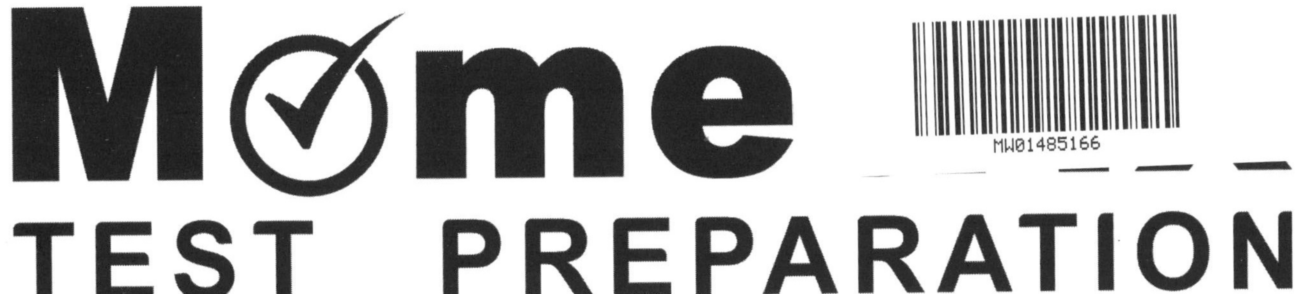


# Nursing Professional Development Exam Secrets Study Guide

Nursing Professional Development Test Review for the Nursing Professional Development Board Certification Test

# Dear Future Exam Success Story

First of all, **THANK YOU** for purchasing Mometrix study materials!

Second, congratulations! You are one of the few determined test-takers who are committed to doing whatever it takes to excel on your exam. **You have come to the right place.** We developed these study materials with one goal in mind: to deliver you the information you need in a format that's concise and easy to use.

In addition to optimizing your guide for the content of the test, we've outlined our recommended steps for breaking down the preparation process into small, attainable goals so you can make sure you stay on track.

We've also analyzed the entire test-taking process, identifying the most common pitfalls and showing how you can overcome them and be ready for any curveball the test throws you.

Standardized testing is one of the biggest obstacles on your road to success, which only increases the importance of doing well in the high-pressure, high-stakes environment of test day. Your results on this test could have a significant impact on your future, and this guide provides the information and practical advice to help you achieve your full potential on test day.

**Your success is our success**

**We would love to hear from you!** If you would like to share the story of your exam success or if you have any questions or comments in regard to our products, please contact us at **800-673-8175** or **support@mometrix.com**.

Thanks again for your business and we wish you continued success!

Sincerely,
The Mometrix Test Preparation Team

**Need more help? Check out our flashcards at:**
**http://MometrixFlashcards.com/NursingProfDev**


Written and edited by the Mometrix Exam Secrets Test Prep Team
Printed in the United States of America

# TABLE OF CONTENTS

# Introduction

**Thank you for purchasing this resource**! You have made the choice to prepare yourself for a test that could have a huge impact on your future, and this guide is designed to help you be fully ready for test day. Obviously, it's important to have a solid understanding of the test material, but you also need to be prepared for the unique environment and stressors of the test, so that you can perform to the best of your abilities.

For this purpose, the first section that appears in this guide is the **Secret Keys**. We've devoted countless hours to meticulously researching what works and what doesn't, and we've boiled down our findings to the five most impactful steps you can take to improve your performance on the test. We start at the beginning with study planning and move through the preparation process, all the way to the testing strategies that will help you get the most out of what you know when you're finally sitting in front of the test.

We recommend that you start preparing for your test as far in advance as possible. However, if you've bought this guide as a last-minute study resource and only have a few days before your test, we recommend that you skip over the first two Secret Keys since they address a long-term study plan.

If you struggle with **test anxiety**, we strongly encourage you to check out our recommendations for how you can overcome it. Test anxiety is a formidable foe, but it can be beaten, and we want to make sure you have the tools you need to defeat it.

# Secret Key #1 – Plan Big, Study Small

There's a lot riding on your performance. If you want to ace this test, you're going to need to keep your skills sharp and the material fresh in your mind. You need a plan that lets you review everything you need to know while still fitting in your schedule. We'll break this strategy down into three categories.

## Information Organization

Start with the information you already have: the official test outline. From this, you can make a complete list of all the concepts you need to cover before the test. Organize these concepts into groups that can be studied together, and create a list of any related vocabulary you need to learn so you can brush up on any difficult terms. You'll want to keep this vocabulary list handy once you actually start studying since you may need to add to it along the way.

## Time Management

Once you have your set of study concepts, decide how to spread them out over the time you have left before the test. Break your study plan into small, clear goals so you have a manageable task for each day and know exactly what you're doing. Then just focus on one small step at a time. When you manage your time this way, you don't need to spend hours at a time studying. Studying a small block of content for a short period each day helps you retain information better and avoid stressing over how much you have left to do. You can relax knowing that you have a plan to cover everything in time. In order for this strategy to be effective though, you have to start studying early and stick to your schedule. Avoid the exhaustion and futility that comes from last-minute cramming!

## Study Environment

The environment you study in has a big impact on your learning. Studying in a coffee shop, while probably more enjoyable, is not likely to be as fruitful as studying in a quiet room. It's important to keep distractions to a minimum. You're only planning to study for a short block of time, so make the most of it. Don't pause to check your phone or get up to find a snack. It's also important to **avoid multitasking**. Research has consistently shown that multitasking will make your studying dramatically less effective. Your study area should also be comfortable and well-lit so you don't have the distraction of straining your eyes or sitting on an uncomfortable chair.

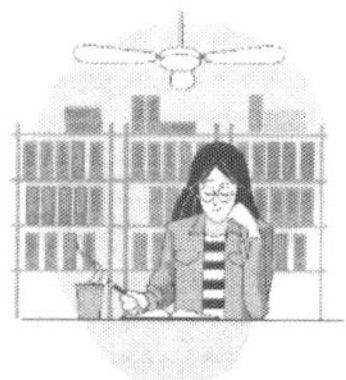

The time of day you study is also important. You want to be rested and alert. Don't wait until just before bedtime. Study when you'll be most likely to comprehend and remember. Even better, if you know what time of day your test will be, set that time aside for study. That way your brain will be used to working on that subject at that specific time and you'll have a better chance of recalling information.

Finally, it can be helpful to team up with others who are studying for the same test. Your actual studying should be done in as isolated an environment as possible, but the work of organizing the information and setting up the study plan can be divided up. In between study sessions, you can discuss with your teammates the concepts that you're all studying and quiz each other on the details. Just be sure that your teammates are as serious about the test as you are. If you find that your study time is being replaced with social time, you might need to find a new team.

# Secret Key #2 – Make Your Studying Count

You're devoting a lot of time and effort to preparing for this test, so you want to be absolutely certain it will pay off. This means doing more than just reading the content and hoping you can remember it on test day. It's important to make every minute of study count. There are two main areas you can focus on to make your studying count.

## Retention

It doesn't matter how much time you study if you can't remember the material. You need to make sure you are retaining the concepts. To check your retention of the information you're learning, try recalling it at later times with minimal prompting. Try carrying around flashcards and glance at one or two from time to time or ask a friend who's also studying for the test to quiz you.

To enhance your retention, look for ways to put the information into practice so that you can apply it rather than simply recalling it. If you're using the information in practical ways, it will be much easier to remember. Similarly, it helps to solidify a concept in your mind if you're not only reading it to yourself but also explaining it to someone else. Ask a friend to let you teach them about a concept you're a little shaky on (or speak aloud to an imaginary audience if necessary). As you try to summarize, define, give examples, and answer your friend's questions, you'll understand the concepts better and they will stay with you longer. Finally, step back for a big picture view and ask yourself how each piece of information fits with the whole subject. When you link the different concepts together and see them working together as a whole, it's easier to remember the individual components.

Finally, practice showing your work on any multi-step problems, even if you're just studying. Writing out each step you take to solve a problem will help solidify the process in your mind, and you'll be more likely to remember it during the test.

## Modality

*Modality* simply refers to the means or method by which you study. Choosing a study modality that fits your own individual learning style is crucial. No two people learn best in exactly the same way, so it's important to know your strengths and use them to your advantage.

For example, if you learn best by visualization, focus on visualizing a concept in your mind and draw an image or a diagram. Try color-coding your notes, illustrating them, or creating symbols that will trigger your mind to recall a learned concept. If you learn best by hearing or discussing information, find a study partner who learns the same way or read aloud to yourself. Think about how to put the information in your own words. Imagine that you are giving a lecture on the topic and record yourself so you can listen to it later.

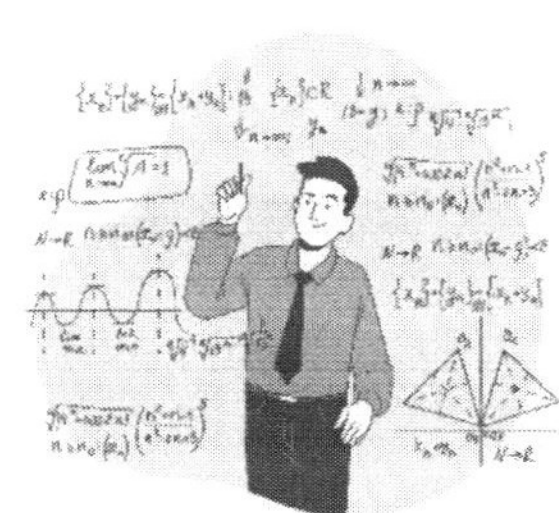

For any learning style, flashcards can be helpful. Organize the information so you can take advantage of spare moments to review. Underline key words or phrases. Use different colors for different categories. Mnemonic devices (such as creating a short list in which every item starts with the same letter) can also help with retention. Find what works best for you and use it to store the information in your mind most effectively and easily.

# Secret Key #3 – Practice the Right Way

Your success on test day depends not only on how many hours you put into preparing, but also on whether you prepared the right way. It's good to check along the way to see if your studying is paying off. One of the most effective ways to do this is by taking practice tests to evaluate your progress. Practice tests are useful because they show exactly where you need to improve. Every time you take a practice test, pay special attention to these three groups of questions:

- The questions you got wrong
- The questions you had to guess on, even if you guessed right
- The questions you found difficult or slow to work through

This will show you exactly what your weak areas are, and where you need to devote more study time. Ask yourself why each of these questions gave you trouble. Was it because you didn't understand the material? Was it because you didn't remember the vocabulary? Do you need more repetitions on this type of question to build speed and confidence? Dig into those questions and figure out how you can strengthen your weak areas as you go back to review the material.

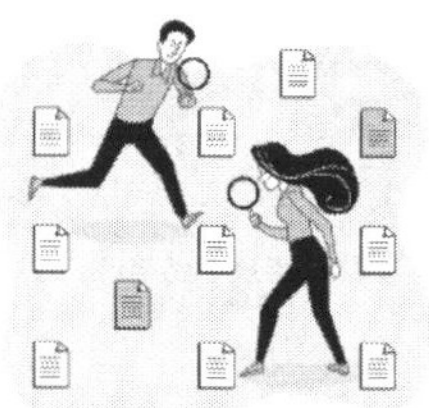

Additionally, many practice tests have a section explaining the answer choices. It can be tempting to read the explanation and think that you now have a good understanding of the concept. However, an explanation likely only covers part of the question's broader context. Even if the explanation makes perfect sense, **go back and investigate** every concept related to the question until you're positive you have a thorough understanding.

As you go along, keep in mind that the practice test is just that: practice. Memorizing these questions and answers will not be very helpful on the actual test because it is unlikely to have any of the same exact questions. If you only know the right answers to the sample questions, you won't be prepared for the real thing. **Study the concepts** until you understand them fully, and then you'll be able to answer any question that shows up on the test.

It's important to wait on the practice tests until you're ready. If you take a test on your first day of study, you may be overwhelmed by the amount of material covered and how much you need to learn. Work up to it gradually.

On test day, you'll need to be prepared for answering questions, managing your time, and using the test-taking strategies you've learned. It's a lot to balance, like a mental marathon that will have a big impact on your future. Like training for a marathon, you'll need to start slowly and work your way up. When test day arrives, you'll be ready.

Start with the strategies you've read in the first two Secret Keys—plan your course and study in the way that works best for you. If you have time, consider using multiple study resources to get different approaches to the same concepts. It can be helpful to see difficult concepts from more than one angle. Then find a good source for practice tests. Many times, the test website will suggest potential study resources or provide sample tests.

## Practice Test Strategy

If you're able to find at least three practice tests, we recommend this strategy:

### Untimed and Open-Book Practice

Take the first test with no time constraints and with your notes and study guide handy. Take your time and focus on applying the strategies you've learned.

### Timed and Open-Book Practice

Take the second practice test open-book as well, but set a timer and practice pacing yourself to finish in time.

### Timed and Closed-Book Practice

Take any other practice tests as if it were test day. Set a timer and put away your study materials. Sit at a table or desk in a quiet room, imagine yourself at the testing center, and answer questions as quickly and accurately as possible.

Keep repeating timed and closed-book tests on a regular basis until you run out of practice tests or it's time for the actual test. Your mind will be ready for the schedule and stress of test day, and you'll be able to focus on recalling the material you've learned.

# Secret Key #4 – Pace Yourself

Once you're fully prepared for the material on the test, your biggest challenge on test day will be managing your time. Just knowing that the clock is ticking can make you panic even if you have plenty of time left. Work on pacing yourself so you can build confidence against the time constraints of the exam. Pacing is a difficult skill to master, especially in a high-pressure environment, so **practice is vital**.

Set time expectations for your pace based on how much time is available. For example, if a section has 60 questions and the time limit is 30 minutes, you know you have to average 30 seconds or less per question in order to answer them all. Although 30 seconds is the hard limit, set 25 seconds per question as your goal, so you reserve extra time to spend on harder questions. When you budget extra time for the harder questions, you no longer have any reason to stress when those questions take longer to answer.

Don't let this time expectation distract you from working through the test at a calm, steady pace, but keep it in mind so you don't spend too much time on any one question. Recognize that taking extra time on one question you don't understand may keep you from answering two that you do understand later in the test. If your time limit for a question is up and you're still not sure of the answer, mark it and move on, and come back to it later if the time and the test format allow. If the testing format doesn't allow you to return to earlier questions, just make an educated guess; then put it out of your mind and move on.

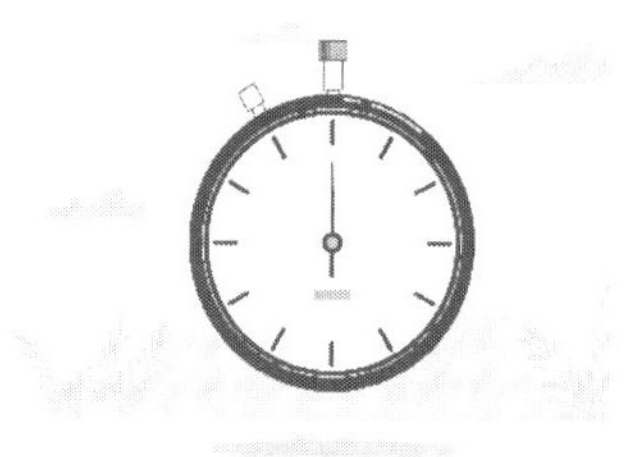

On the easier questions, be careful not to rush. It may seem wise to hurry through them so you have more time for the challenging ones, but it's not worth missing one if you know the concept and just didn't take the time to read the question fully. Work efficiently but make sure you understand the question and have looked at all of the answer choices, since more than one may seem right at first.

Even if you're paying attention to the time, you may find yourself a little behind at some point. You should speed up to get back on track, but do so wisely. Don't panic; just take a few seconds less on each question until you're caught up. Don't guess without thinking, but do look through the answer choices and eliminate any you know are wrong. If you can get down to two choices, it is often worthwhile to guess from those. Once you've chosen an answer, move on and don't dwell on any that you skipped or had to hurry through. If a question was taking too long, chances are it was one of the harder ones, so you weren't as likely to get it right anyway.

On the other hand, if you find yourself getting ahead of schedule, it may be beneficial to slow down a little. The more quickly you work, the more likely you are to make a careless mistake that will affect your score. You've budgeted time for each question, so don't be afraid to spend that time. Practice an efficient but careful pace to get the most out of the time you have.

# Secret Key #5 – Have a Plan for Guessing

When you're taking the test, you may find yourself stuck on a question. Some of the answer choices seem better than others, but you don't see the one answer choice that is obviously correct. What do you do?

The scenario described above is very common, yet most test takers have not effectively prepared for it. Developing and practicing a plan for guessing may be one of the single most effective uses of your time as you get ready for the exam.

In developing your plan for guessing, there are three questions to address:

- When should you start the guessing process?
- How should you narrow down the choices?
- Which answer should you choose?

## When to Start the Guessing Process

Unless your plan for guessing is to select C every time (which, despite its merits, is not what we recommend), you need to leave yourself enough time to apply your answer elimination strategies. Since you have a limited amount of time for each question, that means that if you're going to give yourself the best shot at guessing correctly, you have to decide quickly whether or not you will guess.

Of course, the best-case scenario is that you don't have to guess at all, so first, see if you can answer the question based on your knowledge of the subject and basic reasoning skills. Focus on the key words in the question and try to jog your memory of related topics. Give yourself a chance to bring the knowledge to mind, but once you realize that you don't have (or you can't access) the knowledge you need to answer the question, it's time to start the guessing process.

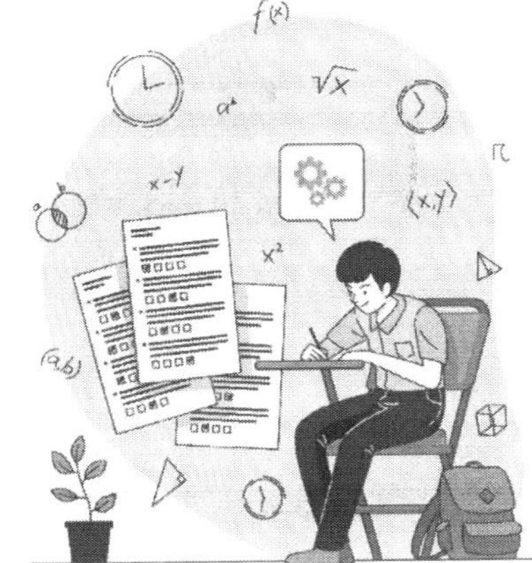

It's almost always better to start the guessing process too early than too late. It only takes a few seconds to remember something and answer the question from knowledge. Carefully eliminating wrong answer choices takes longer. Plus, going through the process of eliminating answer choices can actually help jog your memory.

**Summary**: Start the guessing process as soon as you decide that you can't answer the question based on your knowledge.

## How to Narrow Down the Choices

The next chapter in this book (**Test-Taking Strategies**) includes a wide range of strategies for how to approach questions and how to look for answer choices to eliminate. You will definitely want to read those carefully, practice them, and figure out which ones work best for you. Here though, we're going to address a mindset rather than a particular strategy.

Your odds of guessing an answer correctly depend on how many options you are choosing from.

| **Number of options left** | 5 | 4 | 3 | 2 | 1 |
|---|---|---|---|---|---|
| **Odds of guessing correctly** | 20% | 25% | 33% | 50% | 100% |

You can see from this chart just how valuable it is to be able to eliminate incorrect answers and make an educated guess, but there are two things that many test takers do that cause them to miss out on the benefits of guessing:

- Accidentally eliminating the correct answer
- Selecting an answer based on an impression

We'll look at the first one here, and the second one in the next section.

To avoid accidentally eliminating the correct answer, we recommend a thought exercise called **the $5 challenge**. In this challenge, you only eliminate an answer choice from contention if you are willing to bet $5 on it being wrong. Why $5? Five dollars is a small but not insignificant amount of money. It's an amount you could afford to lose but wouldn't want to throw away. And while losing $5 once might not hurt too much, doing it twenty times will set you back $100. In the same way, each small decision you make—eliminating a choice here, guessing on a question there—won't by itself impact your score very much, but when you put them all together, they can make a big difference. By holding each answer choice elimination decision to a higher standard, you can reduce the risk of accidentally eliminating the correct answer.

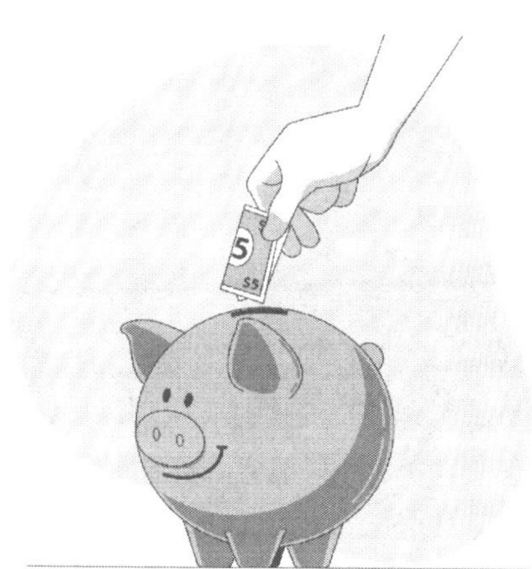

The $5 challenge can also be applied in a positive sense: If you are willing to bet $5 that an answer choice *is* correct, go ahead and mark it as correct.

**Summary**: Only eliminate an answer choice if you are willing to bet $5 that it is wrong.

## Which Answer to Choose

You're taking the test. You've run into a hard question and decided you'll have to guess. You've eliminated all the answer choices you're willing to bet $5 on. Now you have to pick an answer. Why do we even need to talk about this? Why can't you just pick whichever one you feel like when the time comes?

The answer to these questions is that if you don't come into the test with a plan, you'll rely on your impression to select an answer choice, and if you do that, you risk falling into a trap. The test writers know that everyone who takes their test will be guessing on some of the questions, so they intentionally write wrong answer choices to seem plausible. You still have to pick an answer though, and if the wrong answer choices are designed to look right, how can you ever be sure that you're not falling for their trap? The best solution we've found to this dilemma is to take the decision out of your hands entirely. Here is the process we recommend:

**Once you've eliminated any choices that you are confident (willing to bet $5) are wrong, select the first remaining choice as your answer.**

Whether you choose to select the first remaining choice, the second, or the last, the important thing is that you use some preselected standard. Using this approach guarantees that you will not be enticed into selecting an answer choice that looks right, because you are not basing your decision on how the answer choices look.

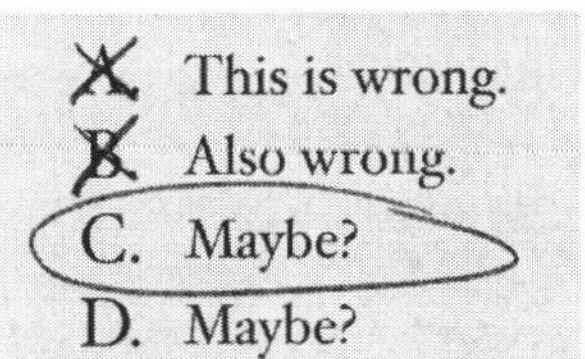


This is not meant to make you question your knowledge. Instead, it is to help you recognize the difference between your knowledge and your impressions. There's a huge difference between thinking an answer is right because of what you know, and thinking an answer is right because it looks or sounds like it should be right.

**Summary**: To ensure that your selection is appropriately random, make a predetermined selection from among all answer choices you have not eliminated.

# Test-Taking Strategies

This section contains a list of test-taking strategies that you may find helpful as you work through the test. By taking what you know and applying logical thought, you can maximize your chances of answering any question correctly!

It is very important to realize that every question is different and every person is different: no single strategy will work on every question, and no single strategy will work for every person. That's why we've included all of them here, so you can try them out and determine which ones work best for different types of questions and which ones work best for you.

## Question Strategies

### ✓ READ CAREFULLY

Read the question and the answer choices carefully. Don't miss the question because you misread the terms. You have plenty of time to read each question thoroughly and make sure you understand what is being asked. Yet a happy medium must be attained, so don't waste too much time. You must read carefully and efficiently.

### ✓ CONTEXTUAL CLUES

Look for contextual clues. If the question includes a word you are not familiar with, look at the immediate context for some indication of what the word might mean. Contextual clues can often give you all the information you need to decipher the meaning of an unfamiliar word. Even if you can't determine the meaning, you may be able to narrow down the possibilities enough to make a solid guess at the answer to the question.

### ✓ PREFIXES

If you're having trouble with a word in the question or answer choices, try dissecting it. Take advantage of every clue that the word might include. Prefixes can be a huge help. Usually, they allow you to determine a basic meaning. *Pre-* means before, *post-* means after, *pro-* is positive, *de-* is negative. From prefixes, you can get an idea of the general meaning of the word and try to put it into context.

### ✓ HEDGE WORDS

Watch out for critical hedge words, such as *likely, may, can, sometimes, often, almost, mostly, usually, generally, rarely,* and *sometimes.* Question writers insert these hedge phrases to cover every possibility. Often an answer choice will be wrong simply because it leaves no room for exception. Be on guard for answer choices that have definitive words such as *exactly* and *always.*

### ✓ SWITCHBACK WORDS

Stay alert for *switchbacks.* These are the words and phrases frequently used to alert you to shifts in thought. The most common switchback words are *but, although,* and *however.* Others include *nevertheless, on the other hand, even though, while, in spite of, despite,* and *regardless of.* Switchback words are important to catch because they can change the direction of the question or an answer choice.

### ☑ Face Value

When in doubt, use common sense. Accept the situation in the problem at face value. Don't read too much into it. These problems will not require you to make wild assumptions. If you have to go beyond creativity and warp time or space in order to have an answer choice fit the question, then you should move on and consider the other answer choices. These are normal problems rooted in reality. The applicable relationship or explanation may not be readily apparent, but it is there for you to figure out. Use your common sense to interpret anything that isn't clear.

## Answer Choice Strategies

### ☑ Answer Selection

The most thorough way to pick an answer choice is to identify and eliminate wrong answers until only one is left, then confirm it is the correct answer. Sometimes an answer choice may immediately seem right, but be careful. The test writers will usually put more than one reasonable answer choice on each question, so take a second to read all of them and make sure that the other choices are not equally obvious. As long as you have time left, it is better to read every answer choice than to pick the first one that looks right without checking the others.

### ☑ Answer Choice Families

An answer choice family consists of two (in rare cases, three) answer choices that are very similar in construction and cannot all be true at the same time. If you see two answer choices that are direct opposites or parallels, one of them is usually the correct answer. For instance, if one answer choice says that quantity $x$ increases and another either says that quantity $x$ decreases (opposite) or says that quantity $y$ increases (parallel), then those answer choices would fall into the same family. An answer choice that doesn't match the construction of the answer choice family is more likely to be incorrect. Most questions will not have answer choice families, but when they do appear, you should be prepared to recognize them.

### ☑ Eliminate Answers

Eliminate answer choices as soon as you realize they are wrong, but make sure you consider all possibilities. If you are eliminating answer choices and realize that the last one you are left with is also wrong, don't panic. Start over and consider each choice again. There may be something you missed the first time that you will realize on the second pass.

### ☑ Avoid Fact Traps

Don't be distracted by an answer choice that is factually true but doesn't answer the question. You are looking for the choice that answers the question. Stay focused on what the question is asking for so you don't accidentally pick an answer that is true but incorrect. Always go back to the question and make sure the answer choice you've selected actually answers the question and is not merely a true statement.

### ☑ Extreme Statements

In general, you should avoid answers that put forth extreme actions as standard practice or proclaim controversial ideas as established fact. An answer choice that states the "process should be used in certain situations, if..." is much more likely to be correct than one that states the "process should be discontinued completely." The first is a calm rational statement and doesn't even make a definitive, uncompromising stance, using a hedge word *if* to provide wiggle room, whereas the second choice is far more extreme.

### ⊘ Benchmark

As you read through the answer choices and you come across one that seems to answer the question well, mentally select that answer choice. This is not your final answer, but it's the one that will help you evaluate the other answer choices. The one that you selected is your benchmark or standard for judging each of the other answer choices. Every other answer choice must be compared to your benchmark. That choice is correct until proven otherwise by another answer choice beating it. If you find a better answer, then that one becomes your new benchmark. Once you've decided that no other choice answers the question as well as your benchmark, you have your final answer.

### ⊘ Predict the Answer

Before you even start looking at the answer choices, it is often best to try to predict the answer. When you come up with the answer on your own, it is easier to avoid distractions and traps because you will know exactly what to look for. The right answer choice is unlikely to be word-for-word what you came up with, but it should be a close match. Even if you are confident that you have the right answer, you should still take the time to read each option before moving on.

## General Strategies

### ⊘ Tough Questions

If you are stumped on a problem or it appears too hard or too difficult, don't waste time. Move on! Remember though, if you can quickly check for obviously incorrect answer choices, your chances of guessing correctly are greatly improved. Before you completely give up, at least try to knock out a couple of possible answers. Eliminate what you can and then guess at the remaining answer choices before moving on.

### ⊘ Check Your Work

Since you will probably not know every term listed and the answer to every question, it is important that you get credit for the ones that you do know. Don't miss any questions through careless mistakes. If at all possible, try to take a second to look back over your answer selection and make sure you've selected the correct answer choice and haven't made a costly careless mistake (such as marking an answer choice that you didn't mean to mark). This quick double check should more than pay for itself in caught mistakes for the time it costs.

### ⊘ Pace Yourself

It's easy to be overwhelmed when you're looking at a page full of questions; your mind is confused and full of random thoughts, and the clock is ticking down faster than you would like. Calm down and maintain the pace that you have set for yourself. Especially as you get down to the last few minutes of the test, don't let the small numbers on the clock make you panic. As long as you are on track by monitoring your pace, you are guaranteed to have time for each question.

### ⊘ Don't Rush

It is very easy to make errors when you are in a hurry. Maintaining a fast pace in answering questions is pointless if it makes you miss questions that you would have gotten right otherwise. Test writers like to include distracting information and wrong answers that seem right. Taking a little extra time to avoid careless mistakes can make all the difference in your test score. Find a pace that allows you to be confident in the answers that you select.

### ⊘ Keep Moving

Panicking will not help you pass the test, so do your best to stay calm and keep moving. Taking deep breaths and going through the answer elimination steps you practiced can help to break through a stress barrier and keep your pace.

## Final Notes

The combination of a solid foundation of content knowledge and the confidence that comes from practicing your plan for applying that knowledge is the key to maximizing your performance on test day. As your foundation of content knowledge is built up and strengthened, you'll find that the strategies included in this chapter become more and more effective in helping you quickly sift through the distractions and traps of the test to isolate the correct answer.

Now that you're preparing to move forward into the test content chapters of this book, be sure to keep your goal in mind. As you read, think about how you will be able to apply this information on the test. If you've already seen sample questions for the test and you have an idea of the question format and style, try to come up with questions of your own that you can answer based on what you're reading. This will give you valuable practice applying your knowledge in the same ways you can expect to on test day.

**Good luck and good studying!**

# Educational Professional Standards

## Theories, Models, and Principles

### Maslow's Hierarchy of Needs

Maslow defined human motivation in terms of needs and wants. His **hierarchy of needs** is classically portrayed as a pyramid sitting on its base divided into horizontal layers. He theorized that, as humans fulfill the needs of one layer, their motivation turns to the layer above. The layers consist of (from bottom to top):

- **Physiological**: The need for air, fluid, food, shelter, warmth, and sleep.
- **Safety**: A safe place to live, a steady job, a society with rules and laws, protection from harm, and insurance or savings for the future.
- **Love/Belonging**: A network consisting of a significant other, family, friends, co-workers, religion, and community.
- **Esteem or self-respect**: The knowledge that you are a person who is successful and worthy of esteem, attention, status, and admiration.
- **Self-actualization**: The acceptance of your life, choices, and situation in life and the empathetic acceptance of others, as well as the feeling of independence and the joy of being able to express yourself freely and competently.

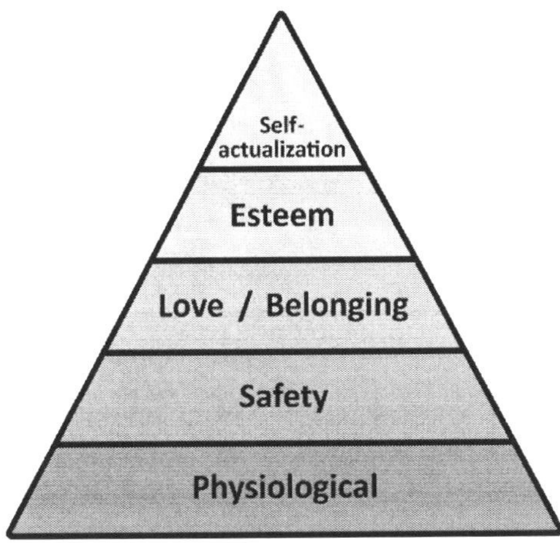


**Review Video: Maslow's Hierarchy of Needs**
Visit mometrix.com/academy and enter code: 461825

### Behaviorist Theory

#### *John B. Watson*

John B. Watson was a behavioral psychologist who built on the experiments of one of the original behaviorists, Ivan Pavlov. Pavlov cultivated his theories from experiments where he conditioned dogs to salivate to different stimuli and developed the **Theory of Behaviorism**. This concept revolves around the use of positive reinforcement to elicit behavioral changes. Watson believed that people could be completely controlled by proper application of reward. Thus, children are rewarded through praise or concrete rewards (points, prizes, computer time, game time, toys) when they successfully carry out a particular behavior, such as toileting. Other theorists believe that this theory ignores the ability of children and adults to act willfully. While using positive reinforcement, negative reinforcement should be avoided as people may respond equally to both. When possible, negative outcomes should be ignored with response only to positive outcomes. Concepts of behaviorism may be combined with other learning theories, such as using models of positive behavior, and then rewarding compliance.

### *B. F. Skinner*

B.F. Skinner developed the **Theory of Radical Behaviorism**, building on the work of Watson, based on the concept that behavior is dependent on the environment and reinforcement. Skinner believed that society influenced the individual and that behavior could be managed by **operant conditioning**. Skinner stated that the individual operates on the environment and encounters stimuli that bring forth a response. Those stimuli that increase the likelihood of a particular response are called reinforcers, and the goal of therapy is to find the appropriate stimuli to reinforce desired behavior. Both positive reinforcement, in which a response is applied, and negative reinforcement, in which a response is removed, are used to encourage or reinforce behavior. Skinner believed that aversive events (such as punishment) weakened behavior but that positive response was most effective. The most important factors in teaching an individual include providing feedback immediately, proceeding from simple to complex in small steps, and providing repetition and positive reinforcement.

## Neuropsychological Theories

Neuropsychological theories of learning focus on different aspects of memory and learning. William James (1890) categorized learning as short-term (primary) and long-term (secondary), with long-term memory involved in processing and storing material. Donald Broadbent (1958) supported this division and described the process in which short-term memories can become long-term memories in his Filter Model of Attention Theory. This theory postulates the presence of a filter between incoming information and short-term memory, allowing people to process more than one piece of information at a time. Neuropsychologists are particularly interested in mapping the areas of the brain involved in learning. Studies also focus on the brain regions that are implicated with different forms of aphasia and dyslexia. For example, developmental dyslexia that results in reading and spelling disability and impaired phonological processing skills and visuoperceptual defects is believed associated with the temporoparietal regions of the dominant hemisphere of the brain. People with impaired phonological processing tend to also have difficulty with verbal memory, which impacts overall memory and learning.

## Psychodynamic Theory

### *Sigmund Freud's Stages of Development*

Sigmund Freud (1900) developed the concept of the unconscious mind and the psychoanalytic approach to therapy. Freud focused on sexuality at different stages of development and viewed the personality as having three parts: the id (basic sexual energy that drives one to seek pleasure), the ego (the realistic part of the personality that tries to find acceptable means of dealing with impulses), and the superego (the part that governs moral and ethical behavior).

Stages include:

- **Oral stage (Birth to 1 year)**: Obsessed with oral activities and must have these needs met for proper psychosocial development, very attached to mother.
- **Anal stage (Ages 1-3)**: Masters toilet training.
- **Phallic stage (Ages 3-6)**: Child focuses on childbirth and differences between the sexes, develops sexual obsession with parent of opposite sex (Oedipal complex—boy drawn to mother; Electra complex—girl drawn to father).

- **Latency stage (Ages 6-11)**: Oedipal or Electra complex wanes, focus is now socialization, begins to gravitate toward the same sex parent to learn appropriate gender roles.
- **Genital stage (Ages 12 and older)**: Puberty, attracted to opposite sex, learns to relate to opposite gender and control sexual drive.

### *Alfred Adler's Individual Psychology*

Alfred Adler developed a theory he referred to as Individual Psychology because he believed that each individual was unique. Adler disagreed with Freud's focus on sex and instead postulated that individuals wanted to maintain control over their lives and that problems arise when a person's self-assertion is limited, resulting in a sense of inferiority. Adler originated the term "inferiority complex," and described striving to overcome the inferiority complex by suppressed the inferiority complex as "superiority complex." Alder's **key concepts** include:

- Inferiority feelings are the source of all human striving.
- Personal growth results from one's attempts to compensate for this inferiority.

Two types of **complexes** exist:

- **Inferiority**: An inability to solve life's problems
- **Superiority**: An exaggerated opinion of one's abilities and accomplishments in an attempt to compensate for an inferiority complex

The goal of life is to strive for superiority. Lifestyle is the unique set of behaviors created to compensate for inferiority and to achieve superiority.

Alder also theorized that **birth order** affects personality:

- **First born**: Happy, secure, and the center of attention until dethroned by the second child; interested in authority and organization
- **Second born**: Born into a more relaxed atmosphere and has the first-born as a model; interested in competition
- **Youngest child**: Pet of the family and may retain a sense of dependency

### *Erik Erikson's Psychosocial Development Model*

Erik Erikson's psychosocial development model covers the life span, focusing on conflicts at each stage and the virtue that is the outcome of finding a balance in the conflict. The first five stages relate to infancy and childhood and the last three stages to adulthood, but childhood development affects later adult development. The stages progress as follows:

- **Trust vs. Mistrust (Birth to 1 year)**: Trust, faith and optimism develop if the needs of warmth, food and love are met. If not, this can result in mistrust.
- **Autonomy vs. Shame/Doubt (Ages 1-3)**: The child desires independence in basic self-care tasks and wants choice. If independence is not encouraged, this can lead to doubt and shame. Independence develops self-control and willpower.
- **Initiative vs. Guilt (Ages 3-6)**: The child engages in self-directed play and starts activities without outside influence. Imaginative play and competition are introduced. This can lead to guilt or direction and purpose based on how this initiative is supportive.
- **Industry vs. Inferiority (Ages 6-12)**: The child values feeling capable and competent, and develops a sense of pride and self-worth. They desire to do what is right and good. Social interactions between peers becomes more important, and comparing achievements can result in feelings of pride or feelings of inferiority if not properly guided.

- **Identity vs. Role Confusion (Ages 12-18)**: Parents, teachers, peers, family members, church, culture, and ethnicity all role model and pressure youth to adopt certain behaviors. The task of adolescents is to discover their own identity.
- **Intimacy vs. Isolation (Ages 18-40)**: Young people learn to commit to another person in a love or family relationship. They learn the behavior required to maintain this relationship.
- **Generativity vs. Stagnation (Ages 40-65)**: Adults have many tasks when they try to find their own interests and niche in the work world. Family, community, and work roles are defined.
- **Integrity vs. Despair (Ages 65+)**: Older people ponder their life experiences to put them into perspective. They learn to accept the aging process and begin to think about their own death.

### *Robert Peck's Stages of Adult Development*

Robert Peck expanded on Erikson's stages of adult development, believing that there were seven important tasks that were required during the last two stages of life:

| Stage | Tasks | Outcomes |
|---|---|---|
| **Middle age** | Valuing wisdom vs. physical powers<br>Socializing vs. sexualizing<br>Cathectic (libidinal energy) flexibility vs. cathectic impoverishment<br>Mental flexibility vs. mental rigidity | Negative outcomes lead to weak relationships, inflexibility, and resistance to change.<br>Positive outcomes lead to strong relationships, flexibility in lifestyle, and adaptability to change. |
| **Older adult-hood** | Ego differentiation vs. work role preoccupation<br>Body transcendence vs. body preoccupation<br>Ego transcendence vs. ego preoccupation | Negative outcomes lead to feelings of loss of identity after retirement, depression, inability to accept bodily/functional changes, and fear of death.<br>Positive outcomes lead to meaningful life after retirement, acceptance of bodily/functional changes, acceptance of death, and feeling that life has been good. |

## Leon Festinger's Theory of Cognitive Dissonance

Leon Festinger's Theory of Cognitive Dissonance states that individuals attempt to escape dissonance and try to avoid inconsistencies between their beliefs and actions. If dissonance occurs, then beliefs and ideas are more likely to change than actions or behavior. Dissonance can be resolved by understanding and attaching less importance to dissonant beliefs, seeking beliefs that are more consonant to outweigh those that are dissonant, or changing beliefs to avoid inconsistencies. Dissonance is especially a concern when the individual is faced with choices and decision making. Because people want to avoid dissonance, they may avoid individuals or situations in which dissonance occurs. A **cognition** is considered a piece of knowledge. When faced with dissonance, the person can:

- Change one cognition to match others or change all to bring them in line.
- Eliminate one cognition or add more to bring about consonance.
- Alter the importance of cognitions.

## Bernard Weiner's Attribution Theory

Bernard Weiner developed the cognitive theory known as Attribution Theory, which focuses on explaining behavior. Weiner suggested that people attempt to attribute cause to behavior, based on three stages: observing behavior, determining that the behavior is intentional, and attributing the behavior to internal or external causes. According to this theory, there are four factors to which achievement can be attributed: individual effort, ability, difficulty of task, and good or bad luck. People often view their own achievement as the result of effort and ability, and the achievements of others as the result of luck. By the same token, people may view personal failures as the result of bad luck and failures of others as the result of lack of effort or ability. Attributions are classified according to three factors: locus of control (internal/external), stability of causes for behavior, and ability to control causes.

## Bandura's Theory of Social Learning

In the 1970s, Bandura proposed the **theory of social learning,** in which he posited that learning develops from observing, organizing, and rehearsing behavior that has been modeled. Bandura believed that people are more likely to adopt the behavior if they value the outcomes, if the outcomes have functional value, and if the person modeling the behavior is similar to the learner and is admired because of status. Behavior is the result of observation of behavioral, environmental, and cognitive interactions. There are **four conditions required for modeling:**

- **Attention**: The degree of attention paid to modeling can depend on many variables (physical, social, and environmental).
- **Retention**: People's ability to retain models depends on symbolic coding, creating mental images, organizing thoughts, and rehearsing (mentally or physically).
- **Reproduction**: The ability to reproduce a model depends on physical and mental capabilities.
- **Motivation**: Motivation may derive from past performances, rewards, or vicarious modeling.

## Theory of Reasoned Action

The Theory of Reasoned Action, developed in 1975 by Martin Fishbein and Icek Ajzen, is based on the idea that the actions people take voluntarily can be predicted according to their personal attitude toward the action and their perceptions of how others will view their doing the action. There are three **basic concepts** to the theory:

- **Attitudes**: These are all of the attitudes about an action, and they may be weighted (some more important than others).
- **Subjective norms**: People are influenced by those in their social realm (family, friends) and their attitudes toward particular actions. The influence may be weighted. For example, the attitude of a spouse may carry more weight than the attitude of a neighbor.
- **Behavioral intention**: The intention to take action is based on weighing attitudes and subjective norms (opinions of others), resulting in a choice to either take an action or avoid the action.

## Theory of Planned Behavior

The Theory of Planned Behavior, by Ajzen, evolved from the Theory of Reasoned Action in 1985 when studies showed that behavioral intention does not necessarily result in action. The Theory of Planned Behavior is more successful in predicting behavior. To the basic concepts of attitudes, subjective norms, and behavioral intentions encompassed by the earlier theory, Ajzen added the concept of **perceived behavioral control**, which relates to the individual's attitudes about self-efficacy and outcomes. Ajzen's theory shows that **beliefs are central**:

- Behavioral beliefs lead to attitudes toward a behavior/action.
- Normative beliefs lead to subjective norms.
- Control beliefs lead to perceived behavioral control.

All of these beliefs interact to influence intention and action. Basically, this theory relates to the person's confidence, based on beliefs and social influence of others, that he or she can actually do an action and that the outcome of this action will be positive. This theory looks at the power of emotions—such as apprehension or fear—when predicting behavior.

## Social Cognitive Theory

Social Cognitive Theory considers that behavior is influenced by the way a person thinks about situations he or she encounters and how he or she then reacts. The issue is whether the person's behavior is more influenced by personality, inborn traits, or the situation. Walter Mischel (1968) found that personality traits and behavior are often at odds; that is, if a person is introverted, studies do not support the idea that the person will spend less time interacting with others. This is a reflection of the person-situation controversy at the heart of Social Cognitive Theory. Mischel noted that just knowing how a person has reacted in one situation cannot necessarily predict how he or she will react in a different situation. Years of various studies have indicated that in order to make predictions about behavior, it is necessary to have information about both the person's personality and the situation. However, situations are interpreted in different ways through personal constructs and personal goals and expectations.

## Cognitive Behavioral Theory

Cognitive Behavioral Theory is a collection of theories rather than one specific theory; however, most are based on the original work of Aaron Beck, who developed cognitive behavioral therapy (CBT). Beck discovered that people often had "automatic thoughts" that occurred related to a personal set of rules. Beck labeled these automatic thoughts as cognitive disorders and identified negative thoughts associated with self, environment, and the world. Cognitive behavioral theories recognize that people have inborn personality traits that interact with situational/environmental factors to influence personality and behavior and to develop a set of core beliefs by which the person interprets events. This is commonly referred to as a nature-nurture viewpoint. If people's core beliefs are in some way distorted or prejudicial, then people may have a misunderstanding of events and may react accordingly, resulting in negative reactions from others. However, these negative reactions tend to reinforce the core beliefs rather than helping people to understand the error in the core beliefs.

## Theory of Cognitive Flexibility

The Theory of Cognitive Flexibility, focusing on the use of interactive technology such as computerized programs, was developed by Spiro, Feltovich, and Coulson (1988). The theory recognizes the complexity and flexibility of learning and suggests that information must be presented from a variety of perspectives and that materials and presentations must be context specific. According to this theory, the primary factor in learning is the ability of the person to construct knowledge. **Basic concepts** include:

- Providing multiple and varying presentations of content. This can include technological presentations (computerized) as well as input from instructors/experts, who can facilitate learning.

- Avoiding oversimplification of content and ensuring that information relates to context.
- Promoting building of knowledge rather than transfer of information. The learner must interact with the material, such as by responding to questions or formulating hypotheses based on information presented, in order to construct his or her own conclusions.
- Interconnecting instructional sources.

## Theory of Brain-Based Learning

The Theory of Brain-Based Learning focuses on understanding the structure of the brain and how the brain functions and stores information in order to develop teaching strategies. Brain-based learning attempts to use research to determine educational delivery. Although there is no singular theory, there is some agreement among proponents on principles. An underlying principle is that the brain and mind are connected rather than separate and that there is a physiological basis for learning. According to brain-based theory, the brain is essentially social, the search for meaning is an innate trait, and learning requires both conscious and unconscious thought processes. Brain-based research has helped to explain learning disabilities, and studies have shown which areas of the brain are involved in different aspects of reading and mathematics, but there is little agreement at present on specific teaching strategies and little supporting evidence, although various approaches have been used, such as studying for short (20-minute) sessions rather than longer periods.

### *Right-Brain/Left-Brain/Whole-Brain*

Roger Sperry demonstrated that the right and left hemispheres of the brain have separate functions that complement each other. Studies indicate that people often have **right brain** (30%) or **left-brain** (70%) dominance, and this affects their preferred learning styles; however, teaching strategies should be aimed at both hemispheres.

| Right-brain individual | Left-brain individual |
|---|---|
| Creative, intuitive thinking. | Critical, analytical thinking. |
| Prefers drawing and manipulating. | Prefers talking and writing. |
| Prefers written instructions. | Prefers verbal instructions. |
| Utilizes images in thought processes. | Utilizes language in thought processes. |
| Has poor organizational skills and is sloppy. | Has good organizational skills and is neat. |
| Enjoys change. | Enjoys stability. |
| Lax about time. | Time-oriented. |
| Prefers geometry to algebra. | Prefers algebra to geometry. |
| Adept at reading body language. | Not adept at reading body language. |

## Teaching Models

Various teaching models exist to facilitate learning in specific learning environments:

| | |
|---|---|
| **Audio/visual tutorials** | Especially effective for supplementary material and for independent study. |
| **Independent study** | Geared toward the needs of the individual and self-paced. Materials may be web-based or paper-based and may include audio-visual materials. |
| **Goal-focused** | Learners presented with a goal and all materials and activities aimed at achieving that goal. |

| | |
|---|---|
| **Guided focus** | Learning takes places outside of formal classroom with materials provided or recommended by instructor. |
| **Anchored** | Activities based on problem solving in relation to realistic case studies. |
| **Collaborative** | Learners work together to complete a learning activity or project. |
| **Project-based** | Learners develop materials (videos, web pages, pamphlets) regarding a topic. |
| **Problem-based** | Learners work in teams to solve problems. |
| **Cognitive apprenticeship** | Instructors model, and learners analyze and apply processes. |
| **Simulations** | Learners actively participate in simulated activities. |
| **Direct instruction** | Instructor-focused presentation. |
| **Cooperative** | Small teams work together through a variety of activities to master a subject, with each member responsible for self-learning and learning of others in the team. |

## LEARNING STYLES

### *KOLB'S LEARNING STYLES INVENTORY*

David Kolb's Learning Styles Inventory classifies student-learning styles based on a learning cycle that includes four stages: concrete experience, reflective observation, abstract conceptualization, and active experimentation. While progressing through all stages is a necessary component of learning, some people prefer a particular style of learning:

- **Accommodative**: Prefers to learn through a combination of concrete experience and active experimentation, solves problems through trial and error, and tends to complete tasks.
- **Assimilative**: Prefers abstract concepts and reflective observation and is more interested in abstract ideas than people and applying ideas.
- **Divergent**: Prefers concrete experience and reflective observations and is imaginative with good ideas and is emotional. Likes working with people.
- **Convergent**: Prefers abstract concepts and active experimentation and prefers dealing with things rather than people.

### *BLOOM'S TAXONOMY*

Bloom's taxonomy outlines behaviors that are necessary for learning and that can be applied to healthcare. The theory describes three types of learning.

**Cognitive**: Learning and gaining intellectual skills to master six categories of effective learning.

- Knowledge
- Comprehension
- Application
- Analysis
- Synthesis
- Evaluation

**Affective**: Recognizing five categories of feelings and values from simple to complex. This is slower to achieve than cognitive learning.

- **Receiving phenomena**: Accepting need to learn
- **Responding to phenomena**: Taking active part in care
- **Valuing**: Understanding value of becoming independent in care
- **Organizing values**: Understanding how surgery/treatment has improved life
- **Internalizing values**: Accepting condition as part of life, being consistent and self-reliant

**Psychomotor**: Mastering seven categories of motor skills necessary for independence. This follows a progression from simple to complex.

- **Perception**: Uses sensory information to learn tasks
- **Set**: Shows willingness to perform tasks
- **Guided response**: Follows directions
- **Mechanism**: Does specific tasks
- **Complex overt response**: Displays competence in self-care
- **Adaptation**: Modifies procedures as needed
- **Origination**: Creatively deals with problems

### *THEORY OF MULTIPLE INTELLIGENCES*

In the 1980s, Howard Gardner developed the Theory of Multiple Intelligences, which states that there are at least seven categories of "intelligences" that people use to comprehend the world around them and to learn. Gardner proposed that teaching that engages multiple intelligences is more effective than teaching focused primarily on linguistic or logical/mathematical intelligences (those most commonly addressed in education). Learners should be assessed to determine their **personal intelligence strengths**, and teaching should address the learners' preferences:

- **Linguistic**: Ability to use and understand language, written or spoken.
- **Logical/mathematical**: Ability to utilize deductive and inductive reasoning, numbers, and abstract thinking.
- **Visuospatial**: Ability to visualize and comprehend spatial dimensions.
- **Body/kinesthetic**: Ability to control physical action.
- **Musical/rhythmic**: Ability to create/appreciate musical forms.
- **Interpersonal**: Ability to communicate and establish relationships with others.
- **Intrapersonal**: Ability to utilize self-knowledge and to be self-aware.

### *VARK*

VARK (**Visual, Aural, Read/Write, Kinesthetic**) utilizes a questionnaire to help people determine their own preferences for learning. The questionnaire has 16 questions with four choices for each question. The questions reflect the four common categories of learning: visual, aural, read/write, and kinesthetic. The person receives four scores, one for each category, so that he or she can better assess areas of strength and weakness. Based on the results, the person is provided the best learning strategies to fit his or her profile. The strategy information includes sections on:

- **Intake**: What the person needs in order to process and learn information, such as written materials, graphs, or demonstrations.
- **SWOT (Study WithOut Tears):** What the person needs to do to make notes and intake into the best form for learning.
- **Output**: What the person needs to do to prepare for examinations.

While VARK is a personal inventory, providing the questionnaire to students is a valuable use of study time, and the information gained can help the nursing professional development specialist develop teaching plans and materials.

### *Dunn and Dunn's Learning Styles Model*

Dunn and Dunn (1967) developed a learning styles model to help instructors identify characteristics that affect learning. According to this model, **five basic stimuli** affect learning:

- **Environmental elements**: Sound, light, temperature, and design.
- **Emotional elements**: Motivation, persistence, responsibility, and structure.
- **Sociological patterns**: Learning alone, presence of authority figure, and flexible learners.
- **Physical elements**: Perceptual strengths (aural, visual, read/write, or kinesthetic), intake (food, drinks), time of day (morning learners, afternoon learners, and evening learners), and mobility (preference for sitting or moving about).
- **Psychological elements**: Global (overview) vs. analytic (step by step), hemispheric preference (right brain vs left brain), and impulsivity vs reflectivity.

The nursing professional development specialist should take into consider all of these stimuli when planning educational offerings. For example, considering light, the room should ideally have some areas with bright lighting and others with low lighting. When considering perceptual strengths, the specialist should vary presentation methods.

### *Myers-Briggs Theory of Personality Types and Learning Preferences*

Based on the work of Carl Jung, **Katherine Briggs** and her daughter **Isabel Briggs Myers** developed a theory of personality types to describe how people look at the world, interact with the world, and learn. This typology is based on four different dichotomous preferences (which result in 16 different personality categories based on where the person lies on these continuums):

| | | |
|---|---|---|
| **Extraversion**: Group interaction, fast paced lessons, experiential learning, Q&A | **vs** | **Introversion**: Independent learning, quiet space, uninterrupted study |
| **Sensing**: Practical, realistic, prefers orderly sequence of details | **vs** | **Intuition**: Imaginative, creative thinker, prefers overview to details |
| **Thinking**: Analytical, fair, low need for harmony, prefers ideas/things to people | **vs** | **Feeling**: Sympathetic, accepting, need for harmony, prefers people to ideas/things |
| **Judging**: Organized, methodical, work oriented, in control of environment | **vs** | **Perceiving**: Open, flexible, play oriented, adapts to the environment |

### *Field Independent and Field-Dependent Perception*

Field-independent and field-dependent perception represent two different styles of cognitive learning based on the studies of Witkin, Oltman, Raskin, and Karp (1971). People are categorized on the basis of the Group Embedded Figures Test (GEFT), which tests how effectively they can identify a simple figure that is inside of a more complex figure. Field-independent learners generally have an internalized frame of reference and perceive themselves as separate from others and the environment, needing little external reinforcement, while field-dependent learners are more externally focused, socially aware, and dependent on others for reinforcement.

| Field-independent learners | Field-dependent learners |
|---|---|
| Unaffected by peer pressure, criticism, and external feedback | Easily affected by peer pressure, criticism, and external feedback |
| Learn best by organizing materials by self | Learn best when materials organized by presenter |
| Impersonal, interested in ideas, self-directed, and prefer lecture format | Social, interested in facts, relate learning to experience, and prefer discussion format |

## Information Process Model of Memory

The information processing model of memory has three primary components: sensory memory, working memory, and long-term memory. Both internal and external processes are involved in the information processing model of memory.

- An **external stimulus** catches the person's attention.
- **Internal processing** occurs involving fleeting (<1 second) sensory memory and encoding.
- The encoded memory is stored in **short-term memory** for up to 30 seconds.
- Strategies facilitate storage of the memory in **long-term memory**, although retrieval may be problematic.
- A response to memory occurs.

When using this model to facilitate learning, it is important to gain the learner's attention and to help the learner to recall previous learning. Repetition and explanation can help to facilitate encoding, and asking for demonstrations of skill and providing feedback can reinforce learning and aid in retrieval.

## Age-Appropriate Teaching Strategies

### *Young Adulthood*

Young adulthood encompasses the years from 20-40 during which people are usually in the cognitive stage of formal operations and psychological stage of intimacy versus isolation. Young adults tend to be autonomous and self-directed and have intrinsic motivation to learn. Their personal experience may enhance or interfere with their learning. Young adults tend to be competency-based leaners who are able to make decisions and analyze critically. The nurse professional development specialist should assess learner motivation and try to identify obstacles to learning and support systems. Teaching strategies include:

- Utilize problem-centered learning.
- Allow people to learn at their own paces and draw on experiential learning.
- Encourage people to participate actively.
- Utilize roleplaying, hands-on practice, and immediate application.
- Keep materials and presentations well organized and clear.
- Recognize the social roles of learners.
- Encourage self-directed learning.
- Focus on health promotion.

### Middle-Aged Adulthood

Middle-aged adulthood encompasses the years from 41-64 during which people are in the cognitive stage of formal operations and the psychological stage of generativity versus self-absorption/stagnation. Middle-aged adults tend to be at the peak of their careers with a well-developed sense of self, although they may have concerns about physical changes. They may explore alternative lifestyles, question achievements, and reexamine values and goals. They may desire change but have confidence in abilities. The nurse professional development specialist should assess learner motivation and try to identify obstacles to learning and support systems. **Teaching strategies** include:

- Be flexible but organized and efficient.
- Assess and recognize potential technology gaps.
- Encourage people to utilize experiential learning.
- Review study skills.
- Relate learning to life concerns.
- Provide reassurance and positive reinforcement.
- Modify approaches for physical disabilities or impairments.

### Older Adulthood

Older adulthood is age 65 and older, during which the person is in the cognitive stage of formal operations and psychological stage of ego integrity versus despair. The nurse professional development specialist should encourage participation, assess coping mechanisms, and provide supplementary materials to reinforce learning. Teaching strategies include:

- Spend a little time getting to know the person so he or she is more relaxed and receptive to learning.
- Determine what information is critical and what is non-essential.
- Evaluate the person's learning style and previous knowledge about the topic.
- Plan for ample time for each session of instruction. Ensure that sessions are closely spaced to reinforce learning.
- Provide the person ample time to practice.
- Allow the person to guide the pace of the session as much as possible and encourage feedback.
- Prepare age-appropriate handouts at accessible reading level and with large-size font.
- Provide materials (pencil, paper) in case the patient wants to make notes.
- Be supportive, patient, and enthusiastic.

## Principles of Adult Learning

Adults have a wealth of life and/or employment experiences. Their attitudes toward education may vary considerably. There are, however, some **principles of adult learning** and typical characteristics of adult learners that the professional development nurse should consider when planning strategies for teaching parents, families, or staff.

- Practical and goal-oriented:
    - Provide overviews or summaries and examples.
    - Use collaborative discussions with problem-solving exercises.
    - Remain organized with the goal in mind.
- Self-directed:
    - Provide active involvement, asking for input.

- Allow different options toward achieving the goal.
  - Give them responsibilities.
- Knowledgeable:
  - Show respect for their life experiences/ education.
  - Validate their knowledge and ask for feedback.
  - Relate new material to information with which they are familiar.
- Relevancy-oriented:
  - Explain how information will be applied.
  - Clearly identify objectives.
- Motivated:
  - Provide certificates of professional advancement and/or continuing education credit for staff when possible.

**Review Video: Adult Learning Processes and Theories**
Visit mometrix.com/academy and enter code: 638453

## Team-Based Learning

Team-based learning involves dividing learners into group, usually of 5-7 learners, to work together on a project or learning experience. Team-based learning usually requires students to meet outside of class in order to prepare some type of project, such as a paper or presentation, although this can pose a problem for adult learners who are employed or have family responsibilities. The instructor should discuss team processes and responsibilities rather than assuming that learners know how to work well in groups. Grading can also be problematic because if one grade is given and some members of a group fail to contribute, then other group members are resentful. One method of dealing with this is to allow team members to grade their fellow group members or assign points to them. Another issue is whether learners will be assigned to the same group for multiple projects or be assigned to different groups.

## Readiness to Learn

The individual's readiness to learn should be assessed because if they are not ready, instruction is of little value. Often readiness is indicated when the individual asks questions or shows and interest in procedures. There are a number of factors related to readiness to learn:

- **Physical factors:** There are a number of physical factors than can affect ability. Manual dexterity may be required to complete a task, and this varies by age and condition. Hearing or vision deficits may impact a person's ability to learn. Complex tasks may be too difficult for some because of weakness or cognitive impairment, and modifications of the environment may be needed. Health status, age, and gender may all impact the ability to learn.
- **Experience:** People's experience with learning can vary widely and is affected by their ability to cope with changes, their personal goals, motivation to learn, and cultural background. People may have widely divergent ideas about what constitutes illness and/or treatment. Lack of English skills may make learning difficult and prevent people from asking questions.
- **Mental/emotional status:** The external support system and internal motivation may impact readiness. Anxiety, fear, or depression about one's condition can make learning very difficult because the patient/family cannot focus on learning, so the nurse must spend time to reassure the patient/family and wait until they are emotionally more receptive.

- **Knowledge/education:** The knowledge base of the individual, their cognitive ability, and their learning styles all affect their readiness to learn. The nurse should always begin by assessing what knowledge the individual already has about their disease, condition, or treatment and then build form that base. People with little medical experience may lack knowledge of basic medical terminology, interfering with their ability and readiness to learn.

## Professional Development Models

Patricia Benner developed the stages of clinical competence for nurses based on the Dreyfus Model of Skill Acquisition in 1984. There are **five stages of clinical competence** for nurses:

1. **Novice**: Has little experience, depends on rules and learned behavior, and is not able to adapt easily.
2. **Advanced beginner**: Has some experience in coping with new situations and is able to formulate some principles of action.
3. **Competent**: Has two to three years of experience and has some mastery of new situations and goals and can cope well but may require time for planning and lack flexibility.
4. **Proficient**: Looks at situations holistically and relies on experience to determine goals and plans and can adapt plans to changing needs and make decisions based on understanding of maxims.
5. **Expert**: Has a wealth of experience to draw from and can provide care intuitively rather than relying on rules and maxims. The nurse is able to understand needs and determine quickly the most effective focus for providing care.

### *Synergy Model*

#### Clinical Ladder

The clinical ladder is often based on the Synergy Model of nurse competencies, which are graded as level 1 (novice), level 3 (competent), and level 5 (expert): clinical judgment, advocacy, caring practices, collaboration, systems thinking, response to diversity, clinical inquiry, and facilitation of learning. The clinical ladder is advancement in the profession of nursing, reflecting the nurse's increased knowledge and skills. Advancement may be through personal initiative, such as when a nurse gets an advanced degree, or may be promoted by the organization, such as when an organization provides incentives and opportunities for advancement. Clinical ladder advancement may be based on:

- **Clinical skills**: Experience, certification in particular skills (such as ECG), training
- **Leadership skills**: Participation in shared governance, committees, mentoring, coaching, supervision
- **Education**: Advance degrees, national certification, continuing education courses, special training
- **Research**: Participation in a journal club, clinical research, presentations, publications
- **Professional development**: Participation in professional organizations, attending conferences, giving presentations

#### Clinical Inquiry

According to the ACCN Synergy model, **clinical inquiry** is a continual process of questioning and evaluating practice in order to provide innovative and outstanding care through application of the results of research and experience. Clinical inquiry requires a desire to acquire new knowledge, openness to accepting advice from mentors and other health and allied professionals, competency in identifying clinical problems, and the ability search the literature for research, critical skills to interpret research findings, and to willingness and ability to design and participate in research. Levels of clinical inquiry include:

- **Level 1:** This nurse professional recognizes problems and seeks advice, follows industry standards and guidelines, and seeks further knowledge.
- **Level 3**: This nurse professional questions industry standards and guidelines as well as current practice and utilizes research and education to improve patient care.
- **Level 5:** This nurse professional is able to deviate from industry standards and guidelines when necessary for the individual patients and utilizes literature review and clinical research to gain knowledge, establish new practices, and improve patient care.

## CRITICAL THINKING

### *STANDARDS OF CRITICAL THINKING*

Paul and Elder (2001) identified a number of standards that must be applied critical thinking:

- **Clarity**: Reasoning should be transmittable from one medium of communication to another, so concepts must be clearly elaborated.
- **Accuracy**: Data and information must be accurate in order to reach the correct conclusion.
- **Precision**: One should anticipate what information others will need and provide detailed and clear information, proceeding from both the general to specific and specific to general.
- **Relevance**: All pertinent data should be collected and insignificant data omitted.
- **Depth**: One should avoid dealing with issues superficially.
- **Breadth**: Situations and data should be considered from various perspectives.
- **Logic**: Assumptions must be valid and conclusions based on evidence.
- **Significance**: Information should be judged on whether it is significant or peripheral.
- **Fairness**: One should be open to new ideas and viewpoints.

### *SKILLS NEEDED FOR CRITICAL THINKING*

Effective critical thinking requires a number of different skills:

| | |
|---|---|
| **Interpretation** | Ability to understand data and explain, knowledge of theories and applications. |
| **Analysis** | Ability to investigate based on objective and subjective data and to consider various methods to solve problems. |
| **Evaluation** | Ability to assess information obtained regarding reliability, credibility, and validity, and to determine if the information is relevant. The person should consider how bias may affect decision making. |
| **Inference** | Ability to arrive at a conclusion based on evidence and sound reasoning. |
| **Explanation** | Ability to explain conclusions and decisions using sound rationale. The person should be able to outline the steps taken to arrive at a conclusion. |
| **Self-regulation** | Ability to monitor personal thinking and to reflect on processes engaged in to reach conclusions. The person should be able to self-correct errors in thought processes. |

### *Steps to Problem Solving*

Problem solving to anticipate or prevent recurrences of dissatisfaction involves arriving at a hypothesis, testing, and assessing the data to determine if the hypothesis holds true. If a problem has arisen, taking steps to resolve the immediate problem is only the first step if recurrence is to be avoided:

1. **Define the issue**: Talk with the patient or family and staff to determine if the problem is related to a failure of communication or other issues, such as culture or religion.
2. **Collect data**: This may mean interviewing additional staff or reviewing documentation, and gaining a variety of perspectives.
3. **Identify important concepts**: Determine if there are issues related to values or beliefs.
4. **Consider reasons for actions**: Distinguish between motivation and intention on the part of all parties to determine the reason for the problem.
5. **Make a decision**: A decision on how to prevent a recurrence of a problem should be based on advocacy and moral agency, reaching the best solution possible for the patient, family, or staff.

## Educational Design Process

### Steps of the Educational Design Process

The first step in designing educational activities is to determine the purpose, such as awareness (changes in Medicare laws), knowledge (new treatments for stroke rehabilitation), safety (use of Hoyer lift), legal issues (sexual harassment), or clinical skills (insertion of PICC lines). The next step is to determine the measurable objectives (desired learner outcomes) and evaluation methods (exam, role playing, return demonstration). Once these are determined, then the content is developed, keeping in mind the knowledge base of the learners. The delivery method may vary widely (lecture, video, internet, podcast, demonstration), depending on the purpose and desired outcomes. Content should be current, well-organized, and easily comprehensible, using aids (such as posters and slide show presentations) as indicated. Learner participation (role playing, discussion, question and answer, return demonstration) should be determined during the development of content as learners engaged in the learning process have better retention. For content involving clinical skills, return demonstrations should be included.

### Assessment of Needs

When designing an education process, one of the most critical elements is a needs assessment to help determine where gaps in knowledge or performance exist. The first step is to identify the target learner and whether it is an individual or a group and, if a group, homogeneous or heterogenous. If interviewing or assessing individuals directly as part of needs assessment, then a private setting is necessary to protect confidentiality. Data may be collected through literature research, questionnaires, pretests, surveys, and observation from the individuals and other healthcare providers. Once needs are identified, they should be prioritized. At this point, resources to support the educational needs should be identified and lesson plans developed along with expected outcomes. The education design process must also take into consideration financial resources of the organization, organizational demands, and time management.

## TEACHING TOOLS

Various teaching tools exist to assist with the teaching process. These must be considered when designing an educational program:

| | |
|---|---|
| **Print materials** | Print materials may be provided before, during, or after class, and can include books, journals, copies of articles, handouts, reference cards, and posters. |
| **Electronics/ Audio-visual** | Computer-assisted learning modules for tablets (e.g., iPad, Nook, Kindle Fire) and audio podcasts are especially valuable for independent study. Videos and audio-recordings may be used independently or to supplement a class presentation. For example, videos may be used for demonstrations if equipment is not available or to show how to use equipment. |
| **Display** | Various types of displays can be used, including whiteboard, electronic whiteboards, flipcharts, or other slide presentations. |
| **Internet resources** | Databases (Cochrane, Medscape Reference, PubMed), NIH/CDC sites, or Medline can provide excellent reference materials. Government sites often offer brochures and pamphlets or guidelines for free download or purchase at low cost. |
| **Equipment** | Various types of medical equipment, mannequins, simulations. |
| **Guest speakers** | Physicians, advance practice nurses, social workers, infection control nurse, administrators, risk managers, and human resources personnel all may serve as guest speakers. |

## PLANNING TYPES OF PROGRAM EVALUATIONS

**Formative evaluations**, which are done while the education program is in progress, must be considered as part of the education design process, and the degree to which the formative evaluations will be utilized to guide or assess the education process must be determined. Formative evaluations that are appropriate should be developed with each lesson plan. For example, a class exercise may be followed by a brief questionnaire asking about the effectiveness of the exercise. If the evaluations are used to guide development of the rest of a course or program, then strict timelines for completing the evaluations and assessing results should be part of the plan.

**Summative evaluations**, which are done at the completion of the education program, should be planned to assess outcomes. As part of the design process, it is important to determine what exactly needs to be evaluated and how best to carry out the assessment to render the needed data.

## LEARNING DOMAINS

### *COGNITIVE DOMAIN*

Learning domains (cognitive, affective, and psychomotor) must also be considered during the educational design process. Much of traditional education is focused toward the cognitive domain of learning, or the thinking domain. Techniques utilized to develop cognitive abilities include lecture, one-on-one instruction, and computer-assisted instruction. Teaching should employ a number of strategies and materials to appeal to different learning styles. For example, audiovisual materials, such as videos, may be particularly helpful to reinforce cognitive learning. When designing educational activities or programs, it is important to consider the knowledge base and prerequisite information that is required in order for learners to participate effectively in the different activities. Additionally, the nursing professional development specialist must consider the time and the amount of repetition that is necessary to bring about short-term and long-term retention. Studies show that distributed practice/education results in better retention than massed; therefore, lessons must be spaced appropriately and reinforcement planned for maximum retention. The cognitive domain is ordered according to increasing complexity: knowledge, comprehension, application, analysis, synthesis, and evaluation.

### *Affective Domain*

The affective domain of learning, or the feeling domain, is often overlooked in traditional education because it relates to the emotional response the learner has to learning rather than cognitive abilities, and cannot be adequately measured but only inferred. The five levels of affective behavior are receiving, responding, valuing, organizing, and characterizing. Teaching strategies that should be included to attend to the affective domain of learning are such activities as role playing, gaming, and simulations, followed by debriefing or reflective exercises. The nursing professional development specialist may also lead group discussions about values, beliefs, and attitudes. Learners may be encouraged to keep journals. Considering the affective domain as part of the education design process is especially important to prepare the learner to make ethical decisions and to help the learner become aware of personal feelings and biases.

### *Psychomotor Domain*

The psychomotor domain of learning, or the skills domain, focuses on fine and gross motor abilities required to carry out tasks. Teaching strategies for the psychomotor domain should focus on mastery of a skill rather than the cognitive and affective domains because psychomotor skills require singular attention. The nursing professional development specialist should avoid interrupting skills practice with questions, such as, "What is the purpose of this step?" as this may negatively impact concentration. Lessons should allow for repeated practice with adequate time to develop mastery. Some skills require little practice while others require extensive practice and periodic relearning, especially if the skill is not frequently used. Skills should generally be practiced in the laboratory environment before used in clinical practice; however, studies also indicate that self-directed practice is as effective as structured. The 5 levels of psychomotor learning in ascending order are imitation, manipulation, precision, articulation, and naturalization.

# Educational Activities

## Developing an Orientation Program

When developing an orientation program, the nursing professional development specialist should first meet with department administrators to gain valuable insight and information, to show respect for their positions and experience, and to gain cooperation. However, the specialist cannot depend solely on the administrators' suggestions but should follow up with various types of needs assessments, including literature research, observation, interviews, surveys, and reviews of similar orientation programs. Expected outcomes should be identified in the process. Some orientation programs are primarily classroom based with reviews of policies, procedures, and equipment, but many nurses feel overwhelmed when orientation ends, especially new graduates who may lack the experience necessary to work autonomously. For that reason, orientation often includes an ongoing mentoring program to provide support for nurses and the opportunity to benefit and learn from the expertise of others. Formal mentoring programs usually establish one-on-one mentoring relationships rather than the more informal mentoring that occurs when one nurse assists another.

## Participating in Nursing Orientation

The nursing professional development specialist's participation in the facility's nursing orientation program for healthcare workers is important because it signals the administrative commitment to performance improvement and staff development. The specialist should clearly outline the following:

- **Area of expertise**: This should include any specialty training, degree, and a discussion of the patient population (age, gender, disease-specific) served.
- **Experience**: The specialist should describe the type and duration of experience related to the area of specialty. New graduates can explain previous (if related) work history and work experience during CNS training.
- **Role in the facility**: The specialist should clearly outline his or her responsibilities and services provided to the facility and the staff, including serving as mentor and/or resource person for staff members.
- **Availability**: Staff members need to know when the specialist is available, including hours and days of work.
- **Methods of contact**: The specialist should provide a telephone number, pager number (if appropriate), and/or an email address.

## In-Service Programs

When developing in-service programs, the nursing professional specialist should develop instructional presentations based on:

- **Required content**: These may be mandated by state or federal regulations or by the organization and must be presented with the required frequency and can include such topics as sexual harassment, CPR, and infection control.
- **Deficiencies**: Educational content should address deficiencies noted in evaluation or accreditation procedures, such as failure to administer aspirin to patients with heart attacks.
- **New developments**: Changes in best practices and new treatments and/or equipment should be presented in in-service so that staff remains current with changes in practice.
- **Local concerns**: In some cases, in-service programs should target issues that affect the local population and about which the staff should be familiar, such as heroin overdoses and Lyme disease.
- **National/Future concerns**: In-service program should anticipate problems that may occur even though they are not evident locally at the present time, such as recognizing and dealing with Zika infections.

## Competency Validation

The first task in competency validation is to select the criteria that will be used to determine competency. Criteria may be selected by review of certification requirements, literature, course content, and job descriptions. The nursing professional development specialist should develop a rubric that lists expected competencies and a range of possible scores (such as 1-4) indicating the degree of competence with explanations for each score. In some cases, if specific tasks are part of the competency validation, then a checklist should be prepared to guide the individual and to ensure that all tasks are completed as part of the individual's evaluation. Then, the person responsible for completing the competency validation should be selected. In some cases, the individual may be asked to do a self-evaluation; otherwise, the competency validation should be completed in collaboration with the individual.

## Preceptor Development

Preceptorship pairs students or novice nurses with those with more experience and knowledge. This is a model for teaching-learning that is increasingly being utilized. While mentoring may entail a long-term relationship, preceptoring is usually a time-limited arrangement related to a term of study, such as a semester, orientation period, or a clinical rotation. The preceptor must balance responsibilities and ensure that he or she is able to provide adequate clinical supervision and guidance to the learner on a daily basis. This may require coordinating schedules and planning carefully to ensure all responsibilities can be met. The preceptor helps the learner to understand his or her impact on the spheres of influence (patient/client, nurse and nurse practice, and organization/system) by including the learner in all activities. The preceptor may engage in shared care as well as direct supervision in order to improve the learner's skills.

## Role Transition

Role transition is moving from one professional level to another (graduate nurse to RN) or from responsibility to another (such as from surgical nurse to oncology nurse). The professional's previous experience must be integrated with new information and a different perception of role. **Problems encountered** in role transition can include:

- Emotional and physical exhaustion and stress
- Professional "bullying" by more experienced staff
- Self-doubt and questioning
- Intrapersonal and interpersonal conflicts
- Lack of adequate mentoring and support
- Disconnection from previous support system

The needs of the individual involved in role transition must be carefully assessed and education provided to allow the person to function in the new role with confidence and effectiveness with adequate time provided for the person to overcome transition shock. A thorough and detailed orientation to the professional role and clinical duties is primary. The individual must be encouraged to express concerns and educational needs and be provided regular feedback and support.

### *Stages of Role Transition*

The stages of role transition are generally thought to occur over the course of 12 months.

| | |
|---|---|
| **Doing** (3-4 months) | The first stage involves transition shock with emotional lability and self-doubt as individuals learn new skills and recognize their limitations. They may be unsure of responsibilities and expectations and not know whom to turn to for assistance and must adjust and accommodate changes. Problem-solving skills are often limited because of lack of experience. |
| **Being** (4-5 months) | The second stage involves transition crisis during which knowledge increases along with self-doubt. Individuals have continued stress but increased awareness of their individual role in health care. They begin to question and examine healthcare issues, searching for answers, and may find themselves placed in clinical positions in which they feel unprepared. |

| | |
|---|---|
| **Knowing** (3-4 months) | The last stage involves acceptance of the new role and recovering from some of the problems and stresses of earlier stages. Individuals begin to separate from earlier support systems and explore and critique their new roles, gaining confidence. |

## Research and Scholarship

The professional development nurse has a responsibility to be involved in research and scholarship. Research must be planned and carried out with standard research methods. All nurses are expected to research and apply evidence-based practices to nursing care. **Clinical research** may be based on observation of patients' needs or lack of adequate research findings or conflicting findings regarding an issue and may involve collaboration with an interdisciplinary group of healthcare providers. **Scholarship** involves not only continuing formal education to an advanced degree but also sharing information gleaned from research, such as through publications of articles in journals and/or books, presentations at conferences, and authoring continuing education courses. Professional development nurses may also develop posters, handouts, videos, and slide shows as part of scholarship activities. Additionally, professional development nurses may serve as instructors in nursing programs and mentors and/or preceptors to nursing students.

## Continuing Education

Continuing education may be required for licensure, for certification, and for employment. Each state board of nursing sets state continuing education requirements. Some states require continuing education for licensure every year, others every 2-5 years, while some may require none. Certification often requires specific types and amounts of continuing education. Some employers may mandate that staff participate in continuing education in addition to licensure and certification requirements. Continuing education providers are approved by the state board, and if the nurse wants to be a provider, the nurse must apply in accordance with state guidelines. In most cases, college/university courses count toward continuing education, usually with 1 semester credit/unit equal to 15 contact hours and one quarter unit equal to 12.5 contact hours. Agencies and organization, such as the American Nurses Association, may be approved providers of continuing education.

## Lifelong Learning and Planning for Academic Progression

**Lifelong learning** is the ongoing pursuit of knowledge often simply for the sake of learning. Lifelong learning is almost always a voluntary type of education in which the individual utilizes a variety of resources—including books, magazines, workshops, conferences, videos, continuing education courses, and academic classes—to stay current in one or more fields of study or just in general knowledge to keep informed. For example, many universities and adult schools now offer programs geared to the interests of older adults.

**Planning for academic progression**, on the other hand, requires more formal education and involves further academic studies in order to advance in one's career. For example, an RN with an AS degree may enroll in a bridge program to receive a BS in nursing and then may work and apply to graduate school to work toward an MS or doctorate degree.

## Clinical Affiliation/Academic Partnerships

The first step in establishing an academic partner or clinical affiliation is to identify a suitable partner whose goals and values match those of the home organization or program. Once a potential partner is identified, the parties involved should explore what a partnership/affiliation will entail and the degree to which the arrangement will be contractual, including how costs will be managed and shared and who will supervise and how that will be carried out. Partnerships may be quite limited, such as when learners observe but do not participate in activities, or extensive, such as when two institutions equally sponsor a nursing program. As part of an agreement, benefits and responsibilities of each party should be clearly outlined, and top-level management should be involved in the process. Information about the partnership/affiliation should be disseminated throughout both organizations/programs.

# Needs Assessment

## Internal Learning Needs Assessment

The nursing professional development specialist can use a number of different methods to assess the **internal educational needs** of healthcare workers:

- Review job descriptions to determine the educational qualifications/ certifications for all different levels of staff to determine what, realistically, they should be expected to know about a particular subject.
- Review job orientation and training materials to determine what staff has already been taught about the subject matter.
- Conduct meetings with staff in different departments to brainstorm areas of concern and potential training needs.
- Meet with team leaders and department heads for their input about the need for education.
- Administer short quizzes to staff asking about standard methods, such as barrier precautions and handwashing, to determine basic knowledge.
- Provide questionnaires to staff to obtain information about their own perceptions of what they know or need to know about the subject matter.
- Make direct observations of staff.

## External Learning Needs Assessment

There are a number of methods to assess **external educational needs**. Using multiple strategies provides the most accurate results:

- Consult with the public health department about community issues, such as rates of HBV, HIV, and TB, to determine shared educational needs.
- Conduct mail surveys either of the general populace or targeted surveys of former patients and families. Mail survey return rates are often low, so a large number of surveys must be prepared.
- Conduct telephone surveys of the same groups, usually with better response and lower costs, but they are time-consuming and may require hiring temporary staff.
- Conduct onsite surveys for both inpatients and clinic patients, including both patients and family members. When surveys are requested by staff directly, return rates are good.
- Conduct interviews for inpatients, clinic patients, and families, giving the chance for people to elaborate but requiring much staff time.

## Gap Analysis

Gap analysis is a method used to determine the steps required to move from a current state or actual performance or situation to a new one or potential performance or situation and the "gap" between the two that requires action or resources. Essentially gap analysis answers the questions "What is our current situation?" and "What do we want it to become?" Gap analysis includes determining the resources and time required to achieve the target goal. **Steps to gap analysis** include:

1. Assessing the current situation and listing important factors, such as performance levels, costs, staffing, and satisfaction, and all processes.
2. Identifying the current outcomes of the processes in place.
3. Identifying the target outcomes for projected processes.
4. Outlining the process required to achieve target outcomes.
5. Identifying the gaps that are present between the current process and goal.
6. Identifying resources and methods to close the gaps.

# Planning and Implementation

## Production of Educational Materials

It is impractical to believe that the nursing professional development specialist can produce all **educational materials**, but careful consideration must be given to a number of issues:

- **Price** ranges from free to hundreds or even thousands of dollars for educational materials, which may be handouts, videos, posters, or entire courses or series of courses available online. The specialist must first consider the budget and then look for materials within those monetary constraints. Government agencies, such as the CDC, often have posters and handouts as well as slide show presentations and videos available for download online at no cost.
- **Quality** varies considerably as well. The specialist should consider the goals and objectives before choosing materials, and the materials should be evaluated to determine if they cover all needed information in a clear and engaging manner.
- **Current relevance** must be considered as well. If material will soon be outdated because of changes in regulations, then it will have to be replaced.

### *Images*

Images help to facilitate learning, and visual enhancement (illustrations, photographs) is common in all types of print and digital media. Visualization as part of the learning process is common but not universal, especially in those with learning disabilities. Images transmit information, and the educator must ensure that the image selected transmits the intended message. While studies show that learning is the same with black and white images as with colored images, most learners prefer colored. However, for print media, color is more expensive. The size of the image must be considered in terms of both cost and use. Important details must be easily discerned. If the image contains words or numbers, these should be easily read. Images are copyrighted, so the educator must consider whether use is for educational purposes and meets requirements of fair use or is for commercial purposes, which may require permission to use the image or payment.

### Handouts, Flyers, and Other Forms of Documentation

Written handouts, flyers, or other forms of documentation are a fixture in classes, but many end up in the wastebasket without ever being used, so thought should be given to providing materials that are useful:

- Handouts that simply copy a slide show presentation or repeat everything in the presentation are less helpful than those that summarize the main points.
- Giving out handouts immediately prior to a discussion ensures that most of the class will be looking at the handout instead of the speaker. Thus, handouts should be placed in a folder or binder and distributed before class so people can peruse them in advance or distributed at the end of class.
- Handouts can be used to provide guidance or worksheets for small group discussions.
- Poster-type handouts (with drawings or pictures) that can be placed on bulletin boards are useful.
- Handouts should be easily readable and not smudged copies of newspaper articles or small print text.

### Reports

A number of issues must be considered in the **design and delivery of reports**:

- **Purpose**: The purpose of the report is primary and should be determined first. For example, the purpose may be to update recipients, gain support, indicate problems, or show progress.
- **Recipients**: Those who need to receive the report must be identified and grouped according to discipline or needs as different individuals or groups may need different reports, some more complex and detailed than others.
- **Delivery mode**: This is the method of delivery, which may include paper document, email, electronic document, spreadsheet, or PDF file.
- **Format**: The format may vary from detailed narratives to simplified graphs and illustrations or some combination. Whenever possible, templates should be utilized. Format should include such considerations as color, font, font size, and white space.
- **Size**: This refers primarily to the length (pages, kilobytes, megabytes) of the report.
- **Frequency**: Reports may be issued at different frequency, depending on the recipient and the purpose.

## Use of Technology in the Design and Delivery of Educational Materials

### Electronic/Audiovisual

A number of issues must be considered when teaching and determining the appropriate electronic/audiovisual materials. The physical environment is a major consideration, especially when using electronic/audiovisual materials:

- First, everyone in the room must be able to hear and see. In a small room, a television or computer screen may suffice, but in a large space, a projection screen must be used.
- Another issue is lighting. Some projectors have low resolution and the lights need to be turned off or dimmed and/or windows covered. Turning lights on and off a dozen times during a presentation can be very distracting. A small portable light at a speaker podium or an alternate presentation can be used.
- Text size for presentations is another issue: slide shows or other presentations that include text must be of sufficient font size to be read from the back of the room.

### *Videos, Videoconferencing, and Teleconferencing*

Videos are a useful adjunct to teaching as they reduce the time needed for one-on-one instruction (increasing cost-effectiveness). Passive presentation of **videos**, such as in the waiting area, has little value, but focused viewing in which the nurse discusses the purpose of the video presentation prior to viewing and then is available for discussion after viewing can be very effective. Patients and/or families are often nervous about learning patient care and are unsure of their abilities, so they may not focus completely when the nurse is presenting information. Allowing the patients/families to watch a video demonstration or explanation first and allowing them to stop or review the video presentation can help them to grasp the fundamentals before they have to apply them, relieving some of the anxiety they may be experiencing. Videos are much more effective than written materials for those with low literacy or poor English skills. The nurse should always be available to answer questions and discuss the material after the patients/families finish viewing.

**Videoconferencing/Teleconferencing** allows for audio and visual collaboration at a distance and can be a valuable tool for education, providing access to experts without the transportation costs. In teleconferencing, students may be at multiple sites while interacting with each other and an instructor.

### *Classroom Response Systems (CRS)*

Electronic classroom response systems (CRS) include the use of clickers to respond to questions or educational content. For example, if an instructor asks the class a question, all students can answer with the clicker, which beams responses wirelessly to a computer, so the instructor can immediately determine if the students understood the question and responded appropriately. This is especially valuable in large groups where quiet students (or those in the back) may have little input into discussions. Additionally, responses can be projected from the computer onto a screen and, in some cases, graphed, so that students are able to see the results of the questions visually. One major advantage to the clicker is that those who might be afraid to answer or are unsure can do so privately. Students using clickers often remain more actively engaged in the learning process.

## Test Construction

### *Essay Questions and Papers*

Utilizing essay questions and assigning papers are effective means of testing of students' organizational skills and creative thinking. They allow students to provide in-depth information and to integrate knowledge from a variety of sources. Essay questions and paper topics are usually less time-consuming to develop than multiple-choice tests on the part of the instructor but require more grading time; additionally, they may take considerably more time for the learner, especially papers that require outside research. One issue is that grading is more subjective and more time-consuming than other testing methods and can be affected by a student's poor grammar and writing skills. Students who speak English as a second language may be at a disadvantage. Ideally, more than one instructor would read and assess the essay questions/papers, but this is often not realistic. The instructor should develop a very clear rubric that indicates the grading criteria.

### *Charts, Drag and Drop, and Fill-In/Short Answers*

**Charts and exhibits** are used in tests to determine the learner's ability to interpret and use data commonly found in patient's health records. For example, lab results may be exhibited and the learner asked to determine which values require intervention. These types of questions can be time-consuming to develop but test the cognitive domain and critical thinking and are often good simulations of actual nursing decision making.

**Drag and drop** test items are often used to match definitions with terms, but a better use is for learners to sequence a series of actions or to set priorities. However, drag and drop items can be confusing to some learners, and the items selected cannot be ambiguous. There should be only one correct ordering of the items.

**Fill-in and short answer** (one or two words) items are often used for questions that require calculations, such as when calculating drop rates or dosages. Only one answer should be possible and a grammatical clue, such as "a" or "an," should be avoided (use "a[n]").

### *Multiple Choice Questions*

Multiple choice questions comprise both a prompt and possible answers. The prompt (stem) may be in the form of a direct question or an incomplete sentence. Usually, 3 or 4 options are provided for answers. Generally, only one answer should be correct. However, in some cases, all answers might be true but the student directed to choose the best or most appropriate answer. The possible answers should be grammatically consistent with the prompt and should be about the same length. The prompt should not contain information that answers another question on the test. The prompt should be written as a positive rather than negative statement, as negative statements may be confusing to learners. All possible answers should seem reasonable. Questions that include "all of the above" or "none of the above" should be avoided as partial knowledge may provide clues. In multiple response/multiple choice tests, several answers may be correct.

### *Return Demonstration*

A return demonstration is given by learners to show mastery of a procedure. This may be done for each step during initial instruction but should eventually include a demonstration of the entire procedure:

- The instructor should ask if the learner has any questions before the demonstration.
- The learner should gather all necessary equipment, using a checklist to ensure that nothing is forgotten.
- The learner should explain the steps. The instructor can prompt: "Can you talk me through this."
- The instructor should avoid interfering if the learner makes a minor mistake, but if the learner appears confused or makes an important error (such as forgetting to apply gloves), the nurse can prompt: "Why don't you look at the checklist to make sure you've done each step."
- The instructor should provide positive feedback occasionally during the procedure: "You've placed the equipment exactly right."
- Upon completion, the instructor and learner should discuss the demonstration and determine if an additional return demonstration is needed.

### *Concept Mapping*

Concept mapping is essentially a visual form of outlining that allows learners to show the relationship of concepts and thereby their ability to think critically and to organize information in a meaningful manner. The instructor can provide the concepts that the learners must map or leave it up to the students to develop a concept map about a specific topic. Concept maps can be done by hand or on the computer. Learners may be asked to explain their concept maps to demonstrate their reasoning. One problem is that concept maps may become very large, and lack of neatness or poor handwriting may influence grading. Learners must receive instruction and practice in developing concept maps and should have clear guidelines about developing the concept map for testing purposes, including the minimum number of items expected on the map.

### *Oral Questioning*

Oral questioning is one of the easiest and least expensive methods of testing, although the questions should be developed carefully in advance and should require critical thinking and judgment instead of focusing only on factual information and rote memory. A decision should be made about whether or not to record (audio or video) the learner responses because if this is not done, then there is no permanent record in the event that the learner feels the score is unfair. Some learners with a fear of public speaking may find answering oral questions very intimidating, so they should have ample practice before testing. The instructor should have clear expectations about the content required for each answer so that the subjective nature of scoring is minimized. The instructor should avoid leading questions and should not interrupt the learner while the learner is answering a question.

### *True/False and Yes/No Questions*

True/False and Yes/No questions are the weakest format and, although frequently utilized, they should be avoided for important testing. Because of the dichotomous choice, the person can effectively obtain 50% by guessing, so if, for example, a student knows only half of the answers (50%) and guesses at the other half and gets half of those correct, the student could ostensibly get 75% (a passing grade) with little actual knowledge. However, true/false and yes/no questions may be used effectively for quick assessment purposes at the end of a lesson. When writing true/false and yes/no questions, the instructor should write a clear statement that the learner must judge and should avoid questions that contain negatives (no, not) as these are often confusing for learners. One way to improve these questions is to require the learner to explain the reason for the answer.

### *Ordering Items and Writing Directions*

After test items are written, the next step is to actually construct the test by placing the test items in order. Tests often contain different types of questions, so they should be organized by type, such as all multiple choice grouped. Then, within the group, the questions should be ordered according to difficulty, with the easiest questions first and most difficult last because this ordering helps learners to gain confidence. Additionally, the groupings should be ordered according to difficulty with the easiest format (true/false and yes/no) first and the most difficult (essay questions) last.

Directions should clearly express what is needed for the students, such as "provide answer to one decimal point" or "respond with one word answer." The time limit for the test should be stated. For ease of grading, the method of responding to questions should be indicated: "Mark correct answer with an X." The value assigned to each type of item should be stated so that students know where to focus the most attention.

### *Item Analysis*

Item analysis is the process of determining whether or not a test item discriminates those who are learners from non-learners. Item analysis includes:

- **Difficulty index (*P* value):** This reflects the percentage of students who answer an item correctly. For example, if 100% of students answer correctly, the difficulty index (*P* value) is 1.0, and this usually means that the question is too easy to differentiate between learners and non-learners, so a target difficulty index is usually in the range of 0.7-0.8.
- **Discrimination**: This refers to whether the test item can differentiate those who know the content from those who do not, comparing answers to items on the test to the overall test score (point biserial correlation). Test items that discriminate well have a point biserial correlation of 0.3 or better, although this is affected by the difficulty index.

- **Distractor evaluation**: Each distractor (such as in multiple choice questions) should be evaluated to determine how often it is selected. For example, if one distractor is rarely or never selected (point biserial correlation of 0.0), then the distractor is probably not plausible and should be revised.
- **Reliability coefficient**: This evaluates whether a test taken twice produces similar results and determines whether a test is completely unreliable (coefficient of 0.0) or 100% reliable (coefficient of 1.0). Standardized tests that have undergone rigorous evaluation should have a reliability coefficient of 0.9 or greater, but classroom tests usually range from 0.7-0.9 with scores below this suggesting that some items should be replaced or revised.

While item analysis can be done manually, computer programs are available that can provide accurate item analysis.

#### *Validation*

Validation ensures that the test actually measures that which is intended and has accuracy (measures objectives precisely), utility (provides formative and summative results), and relevance (provides meaningful results). The validity of a test is determined in relation to a reference group (the group that will be tested). **Categories of validity** include:

- **Content-related**: The test should be reviewed to ensure it includes questions that represent all content.
- **Criterion-related**: The scores on the test should correlate with other forms of measurement, so it can be used to predict success in other measures, such as certification tests (predictive validity). Scores of a test may be assessed in relation to scores on a test that is already validated (concurrent validity). High scores should correlate with high degree of clinical competence
- **Construct-related**: The test should be evaluated to determine the degree to which outside variables affect outcomes, such as personal experience and IQ.

### Just-In-Time Educational Programs

Just-in-time presentations are those presented when the learner or learners need to use the information. For example, if teaching learners to access data in a new computerized system, a supportive overview of the system and its purpose may be given right before hands-on practice along with basic instructions about use. However, only when the learners need to access data is the presentation about data access provided. This allows the learners to immediately draw on what they are learning without the typical memory loss that occurs when people are trying to retrieve information they learned at an earlier time. Just-in-time presentations are especially useful with low complex procedural information that helps people to learn to master a specific task. A training session may include both supportive information given immediately prior to practice and just-in-time presentations interspersed throughout the session.

### Rapid Deployment of Educational Programs

Rapid deployment of educational programs is necessary at times, such as the response needed to train healthcare providers on caring for patients with Ebola or COVID-19 infection. The first step when a need becomes clear is to conduct a risk analysis and needs assessment that involves setting parameters, collecting data, analyzing results, and establishing priorities. This process usually takes at least 3-5 days. Once needs are outlined, then key stakeholders and resources must be identified and a plan for rapid deployment developed. The logistics of rapid deployment must be considered, including the need for educators, materials, and space. Funding is often the primary stumbling block to rapid deployment, so addressing this concern must be a priority. Lack of funding, in some cases, results in modifying original plans so that critical information can be covered at lower cost.

### Issues Related to the Learning Environment

The learning environment can influence student's learning and perceptions, so a number of issues must be considered:

- **Room size**: The size should be appropriate for the number of learners and the equipment or materials. If the room is too small, learners will feel crowded and may be distracted, but a space that is too large can also be uncomfortable.
- **Room configuration**: If the instructor wants students to work in groups or engage in discussion, then seating bolted to the floor in rows is not conducive to this type of interaction. Some types of learning activities work best with tables and chairs, so this is a consideration.
- **Temperature**: The learning environment should be maintained at a comfortable temperature. It is usually better for the temperature to be slightly cool than too hot because it is easier to compensate for a cool temperature and learners are likely to be more alert than in a hot environment.
- **Lighting**: Lighting must be adequate for the class activities.
- **Technology**: The room should provide/support needed technology.

### Teaching Approaches

There are many approaches to teaching, and the nursing professional development specialist must prepare, present, and coordinate a wide range of educational workshops, lectures, discussions, and one-on-one instructions on a variety of infection control topics. Planning time for classes should be made as part of the infection control plan, but allow for flexibility to contend with unexpected needs. All types of classes will be needed, depending upon the purpose and material:

- **Educational workshops** are usually conducted with small groups, allowing for maximal participation, and are especially good for demonstrations and practice sessions.
- **Lectures** are often used for more academic or detailed information that may include questions and answers but limits discussion. An effective lecture should include some audiovisual support.
- **Discussions** are best with small groups so that people can actively participate. This is a good for problem solving.
- **One-on-one instruction** is especially helpful for targeted instruction in procedures for individuals.
- **Computer/Internet modules** are good for independent learners.

### Adapting Presentations to Various Audiences

The nursing professional development specialist may need to adapt a presentation to various audiences. The specialist must consider many different factors, including characteristics of the audience, such as age, lifestyle, beliefs, education, occupation, religion, gender, and sexual orientation. Adapting the presentation may result in a change in the language of the presentation (for example, avoiding medical jargon for a non-medical audience), a change in the duration of the presentation or parts of the presentation, and a change in the manner of presentation. For example, a data-heavy presentation might be appropriate for administrators but not for other staff members. Illustrations and images may need to be modified or changed. Examples should be tailored to the audience whenever possible.

## Meeting Content and Scheduling Needs

The nursing professional development specialist should consider the **length, type, and timing of activities** needed to cover the material and whether activities will be scheduled during working hours or outside of working hours and whether staff members receive overtime pay or time off to compensate, because these factors impact scheduling. The day shift (8 AM to 4 PM) is usually the most staff intensive, so scheduling training from 3-4 PM is often the most cost-effective decision because fewer people need to be paid for overtime, and there is less disruption in normal working schedules. Additionally, mornings are a busy time because of physician visits, treatments, and procedures, while late afternoon tends to be freer of disruptions. Training sessions of 1 hour are usually optimal unless training is scheduled for workers' off days. Scheduling multiple training sessions at different times allows more flexibility. The length of the activity also depends on the type, which can include lecture, hands-on practice, video, computer-assisted, or clinical practice.

## High- and Low-Fidelity Simulations

**High-fidelity simulations** are those that use real and/or realistic equipment and materials as part of learning. This can include electrocardiogram (ECG) machines, mannequins, or specialized equipment used in the work environment, so that the learners can actually practice the tasks or procedures that they will carry out as part of their job functions. High-fidelity simulations are often the most helpful for the learner but are also the most costly because equipment may need to be dedicated for learner use. Additionally, training that involves practice and assessment of performance is often more time-consuming.

**Low-fidelity simulations** rely on verbal, print, video, or audio descriptions, and often involve discussion of potential actions rather than actual practice. Thus, learners may be presented with a case study or scenario with specific problems and be asked to describe the process for dealing with the problems. Low-fidelity simulations are less expensive and can usually be completed more quickly, but evaluation may not adequately measure clinical expertise.

## Presentation Styles

### *Formal vs. Informal Presentations*

**Formal presentations** are planned in advance and usually follow an outline or agenda. The language is often more formal, and the audience distance is usually greater. For example, the presenter is usually standing at the front of the room, behind a podium, or on a stage. Formal presentations are often supported by software presentations, videos, or other materials. Audience participation is usually more limited and may include no participation or a short question and answer period.

**Informal presentations** are most often delivered to small groups in an informal setting, such as those sitting around a table. Informal presentations are often impromptu and involve audience participation, often with a free flow of questions and answers during the presentation. While informal presentations may be planned or unplanned, they are usually presented with informal language and not supported by presentation software or other technology, although the presenter may provide handouts.

### *ARCS Model*

John Keller's (1987) ARCS model for creating a motivating learning environment focuses on developing motivational strategies as part of instructional design. Motivational strategies are essential, especially when dealing with learners who lack motivation to learn. Instructors can rarely rely on intrinsic motivation alone and must consider extrinsic motivational techniques. The ARCS model includes the **four key elements** that Keller believed are essential for sustaining motivation in learners:

- **Attention**: Strategies include use of case studies, active participation, humor, comparisons, opposing ideas, and variable teaching strategies. Gaining attention may be done by perceptual arousal (surprise, uncertainty) or inquiry arousal (questioning).
- **Relevance**: Learners' experience, usefulness (current and future), matching personal needs, and choices.
- **Confidence**: Learning requirements, difficulty level, learner expectations, and sense of accomplishment.
- **Satisfaction**: Timely utilization of new skills, rewards, praise (while avoiding patronizing the learner by over-rewarding), and self-evaluation.

### *Additional Presentation Styles*

Additional presentation styles include:

- **Storyteller**: This presenter makes an emotional connection with the audience and utilizes narratives and personal stories to transmit information. However, this presentation style may not be well suited for conveying data, and learners frequently interrupt the presentation with questions and comments, so it can be difficult to maintain a focus.
- **Coach**: This presenter facilitates learning by engaging the audience and encouraging them to come up with solutions and information. Presentations are learner-focused.
- **Teacher**: This presenter focuses on presenting facts and information and providing explanations. Presentations are usually organized and linear and allow for few interruptions. Presentations are presenter-focused.
- **Closer**: This presenter does not like to waste time and gets to the point rapidly. While this type of presentation is efficient and takes less time than others, it may seem too abrupt to some learners and often does not allow for exchange of ideas.

## Selecting Appropriate Teaching and Learning Modalities

### *Debriefing*

Debriefing involves both reflective observation and abstract conceptualization. That is, the learner reflects back on an experience and attempts to find meaning from that experience. The nursing professional development specialist should facilitate reflection through observation and questioning about what the learner observed, felt, heard, smelled, and touched. The specialist should guide learners rather than lecture them. Debriefing is commonly used after role playing to help the learners determine if the role playing was realistic and problems handled appropriately. Debriefing is also commonly used after simulations in order to review the learners' actions and understanding of the problems encountered and to allow them to come up with alternate courses of action when appropriate. Debriefing may also be utilized when errors or problems occur to help those involved determine the cause and how the errors or problems could have been avoided.

### *Narrative*

Narrative pedagogy is an approach to nursing education based on nine themes described by Nancy Diekelmann (2001): gathering, creating places, assembling, staying, caring, interpreting, presenting, preserving, and questioning. Teaching and learning focus on shared experiences and questioning to promote thinking rather than to find a definitive answer. For example, the teacher may provide a narrative example (story) in which there are two possible solutions and ask the learners to determine which solution they would choose and to describe their thought processes, explaining how they arrived at their answers. Narrative pedagogy encourages the learner to look at situations from many different perspectives. The teacher's role is not to answer questions but to encourage persistent questioning. Case studies are commonly used to facilitate learning. Narrative pedagogy may be the focus of an entire nursing program or may be used as an educational tool in some circumstances.

### *Reflective Practice*

Reflective practice is an approach to learning that involves reflecting on a situation or problem in order to find answers or solutions. While reflective observation is part of debriefing, reflective practice is an ongoing process. Various models of reflective practice exist, but all are similar to the **original steps** outlined by John Dewey (1933):

1. Try to get a sense and understanding of the problem faced.
2. Make relevant observations about the problem.
3. Reach a conclusion.
4. Test the conclusion.

Learners are encouraged to identify their feelings, draw on personal experiences, and consider alternative solutions. Questioning and feedback are central to reflective practice and help learners learn to recognize their strengths and weaknesses. Learners are encouraged to seek feedback from many sources. In practice, various approaches are utilized to encourage reflective practice. These can include keeping journals or clinical logs and having group discussions.

# Evaluation Process and Outcomes

## Models of Evaluation

### *CIPP Model*

The CIPP model, a decision-oriented assessment model, is most appropriate to measure the strengths and weaknesses of a program, to identify the needs of a target population, and to identify options. It is based on four different categories of assessments:

- **Context**: Identifies the target population and assesses the population's specific needs as well as weaknesses and strengths.
- **Input**: Evaluates the capabilities of the system, program strategies, plans, and budgets.
- **Process**: Assesses any defects in design or implementation that may pose problems and provides feedback regarding progress.
- **Product**: Assesses outcomes in relation to objectives and transportability to other programs.

CIPP provides information to those in the position to make decisions, such as administrators, about what changes are necessary for a program, how they can be achieved, what is being done, and how successful have changes been.

### *Utilization Focused Evaluations*

Utilization-focused evaluation is evaluation that is carried out for a specific purpose regarding activities, characteristics, and outcomes of organizations or programs. The evaluation is carried out in order to make decisions and judgments, to improve effectiveness, to make future plans, and to provide specific information. The evaluation methods depend on the context and situation. The first step in the evaluation usually entails bringing together key stakeholders to discuss the context in order to decide the focus of the evaluation. Evaluation should be utilized in every stage of development and should include both formative and summative evaluations. The evaluation process looks at impact, process, decision making, and knowledge either individually or simultaneously so the evaluation can remain quite focused or more holistic. Stakeholders should be encouraged to participate so that they see the value of the evaluation process and help to interpret the results.

### *Responsive Evaluations*

Responsive evaluation is a primarily qualitative evaluation that is based on the claims, concerns, and issues of stakeholders, both internal and external. The design of the evaluation emerges from dialogue with and among stakeholders. These dialogues may or may not lead to consensus, but questions should emerge. Stakeholders should meet for dialogue in homogenous groups first and then, as much as possible, heterogenous groups so that concerns can be shared by those from different perspectives. The evaluation should focus on controversies and seek to answer the questions that arise regarding problems. Evaluation techniques may include interviews, participative observations, and document analysis. Measurable indicators, data sources, and data collection methods should be identified and designed to answer specific questions. Responsive evaluations tend to focus on activities and social aspects of a program, attempting to find solutions to problems and identify merits.

### *Ethnographic Evaluations*

Ethnographic evaluation is a qualitative method in which the evaluator is a participant-observer over an extended period of time, watching and listening and gathering data in order to facilitate decision making. Ethnographic evaluation is based on the field of ethnography, which focuses on culture and customs of individuals and groups. Ethnographic evaluation stresses the importance of developing rapport and positive relationships so that the evaluator can ask questions and explore ideas. Various methods are used for ethnographic evaluation, including participant observations and in-depth interviewing of key informants at all levels in an organization. This allows acquisition of contextual information, such as social, political, and cultural influences. Findings are triangulated; that is, they are cross-checked with other findings to ensure that they are consistent. The evaluator should undergo self-examination to determine if biases, values, or belief system have affected conclusions.

### *Multilevel Evaluations*

Multilevel evaluation assesses an organization or program at different levels and is dependent on nested (separate but part of broader) data. For example, data about learners may be nested according to healthcare provider, disease, HMO, age, or various other factors. Data about providers may be nested according to the healthcare system, the geographic area, the specialty, or other factors. The **three primary levels** include:

- **Case level**: Evaluates specific details about an organization/program, group, or individuals. This type of evaluation may help to determine the effectiveness of an organization/program but may be affected by bias.
- **System level**: Evaluates the overall processes of an organization/program and responses. This type of evaluation may show change over time and uses both primary and secondary data.
- **Social level**: Evaluates the effect the organization/program has on society and the environment. This type of evaluation may involve comparisons with other organizations/programs.

## Developing and Conducting Formative Evaluations

Formative evaluations are process evaluations in that they are conducted during the process of learning in order to determine the effectiveness of teaching and learning and progress toward expected outcomes. Formative evaluations, which are generally qualitative, are also used to make adjustments to teaching. Separate funding or time is rarely provided for formative evaluations as they are considered part of the role of teaching. Evaluations should be as non-intrusive as possible. Formative evaluations tend to focus on parts of the education program (such as one lesson or activity) rather than its entirety. Formative evaluations may be proactive, clarifying, interactive, or monitoring. Numerous approaches are utilized, including questionnaires, observations, budget review, time tracking, focus groups (with or without the ORID [observation, reflection, insights, decision] process), and literature review. Formative evaluations should involve multiple stakeholders and different types of evaluation tools to prevent bias.

## Developing and Conducting Summative Evaluations

Summative evaluations (outcomes evaluations) are conducted at the end of a course or program to provide information about effectiveness and outcomes. Summative evaluations, for example, may be used to determine a learner's course grade at the end of a semester. Summative evaluations are usually planned and budgeted for and generally require more planning and expertise to carry out in order for the data collected to have validity. Summative evaluations tend to be objective and quantitative, although qualitative assessments, such as through focus groups and interviews, can provide valuable insight. Methods of quantitative assessment may include questionnaires, surveys, metering (monitoring the consumption of resources), budget review, and various measures of data. When selecting evaluation tools, the nursing professional development specialist should carefully consider the outcomes that need to be evaluated. For example, if return on investment is the concern, then learner satisfaction surveys are of little use.

# Continuing Education Accreditation

## Continuing Education Process

In order to provide continuing education hours, the nursing professional development specialist must provide content through an accredited provider of approved continuing nursing education (CNE) or continuing medical education (CME). The continuing education hours may be sponsored by an organization, agency, or educational institution that is accredited by or approved by the ANCC, ACCME, ACPE, or Commission of Dietetic Registration. The hours may also be provided through an accepted agency, such as the ANA, APA, ENA, and APNA. Individual states may have separate accreditation requirements for continuing education providers. The Accreditation Council for Continuing Medical Education (ACCME), the Accreditation Council for Pharmacy Education (ACPE), and the American Nurses Credentialing Center (ANCC) have a Joint Accreditation program so organizations can simultaneously apply for accreditation as continuing education providers of nursing, medical, and pharmacy continuing education.

## Requirements and Calculation of Contact Hours

Requirements for continuing education vary according to professional status and the licensing state. In order to renew an RN license, states require various numbers of continuing education contact hours. For example, Colorado requires none and California requires 30 hours every 2 years. Advance practice nurses often have additional state requirements as well as requirements for recertification by the certifying organization. In some cases, specific course content is required, such as hours in pharmacology. The nursing professional development specialist must complete 30 contact hours in the 3 years prior to original certification and 75 contact hours every 5 years in order to recertify. When calculating continuing education hours, 1 contact hour generally equals 60 minutes and 1 CEU equals 10 contact hours. One academic semester hour equals 15 contact hours; and one academic quarter hour equals 12.5 contact hours.

## Professional Roles in Continuing Education

### *Approvers and Providers*

The ANCC has an accreditation program for both approvers and providers of continuing education. Both approvers and providers must fill out extensive applications and provide narrative documentation and undergo a virtual visit as part of the accreditation process.

- **Approvers** are organizations that have demonstrated the ability and established standards to approve other organizations or individuals that provide continuing nursing education. These approver units (AUs) operate separately within eligible organizations, such as the ANA and state nurses associations. Once accredited, AUs approve CNE activities of accredited providers. AUs must have a nurse peer-review leader.
- **Providers** are those organizations that are accredited and have met standards for providing quality continuing nursing education. These provider units (PUs) must be able to plan, implement, and evaluate CNE activities. PUs must have a lead nurse planner. PUs may be separate organizations or separate units within larger organizations.

### *Content Experts*

Content experts are nurses with ANCC certification who are experts in their field, want to contribute, and have a leadership role in the ANCC. Application forms are available online for both national and international positions. **Content expert positions** include:

- **Appraisers**: These are nurses with specialty certifications who evaluate portfolios of applicants to determine if they meet requirements.
- **Content expert panels**: CEPs review certification tests on an ongoing basis and develop new tests. CEPs are also charged with role delineation studies every 3 years as part of test development. CEPs serve for a 4-year term and meet for 2- to 3-day meetings 2-3 times a year.
- **Item writers**: These nurses write the actual questions that are used on certification exams.
- **External validation committee**: These nurses complete an online survey (which should not take more than 3 hours to finish) regarding proposals for performance, tasks, and knowledge.
- **Standard setting panel**: These nurses set standards for newly developed certification programs and updated tests. The person must attend a one-time 2-day meeting.

### *Planners and Presenters*

Planners and presenters of continuing nursing education (CNE) are those that actually develop and present continuing education materials and courses that have been approved through a provider unit. Planners evaluate needs assessments to ensure that content meets ANCC provider design criteria. Submission requirements to provider units (PUs) may vary somewhat from one state and organization to another, but generally the course is submitted to the PU for approval and the number of contact hours determined. Presenters are usually nurses but not always. For example, a nutritionist may present information about diet and nutrition; however, if the CNE is about nursing itself, then the content must be presented by a nurse. Presenters are generally licensed and considered experts in the field of presentation. Presenters may present CNEs in face-to-face presentation, but they may also write material that is presented in various formats: written, audio, video, videoconferencing.

### *Managing Continuing Education Credits*

There are a number of aspects to managing the process for continuing nursing education credits. When a learner registers for continuing nursing education, the number of contact hours that will be earned and the requirements (hours of participation, testing) should be outlined. In most cases, the person will receive a certificate upon completion, and it is the individual's responsibility to maintain the certificate as proof of participation through the required state licensing or certification period. However, the presenter must also maintain records, usually for a period of at least 5 years, but this may vary from state to state. Because the records contain personal identifying information, they must be maintained securely. In most cases, presenters now submit data about participants directly to state licensing boards and may also submit data to certifying agencies, simplifying record keeping for participants.

### Evaluating Activities for Continuing Education Credits

When evaluating activities for continuing education credits, the activities should first be evaluated to determine if they meet the ANCC provider design criteria. Continuing education should:

- Address gaps in professional practice.
- Include a nurse planner in the planning process.
- Be based on needs assessment.
- Identify one or more learning outcomes.
- Use appropriate teaching strategies.
- Base information on evidence-based practice.
- Evaluate learning outcomes.
- Be free of commercial influence.

The nurse planner should determine what the target audience is for the CNE, and develop the learning outcomes. Educational content may be selected by the nurse planner or other presenter, but the nurse planner is responsible for ensuring content is evidence-based and involves learner engagement.

# Leadership

## Leadership Principles

### Types of Nursing Decision Making

Types of decision making utilized by the nurse include the following:

| | |
|---|---|
| **Assessing** | A decision about when and how to conduct an assessment. |
| **Communicative** | A decision about how information will be transmitted or received. |
| **Diagnostic** | A decision based on clinical signs and symptoms and nursing evaluation. |
| **Experiential** | A decision based on integration of knowledge, evaluation, and experience. |
| **Informative** | A decision to seek information to further knowledge. |
| **Interventional** | A decision selecting one intervention from various options. |
| **Preventive** | A decision based on which intervention is most likely to prevent a negative outcome. |
| **Referring** | A decision about which professional healthcare provider or services a patient should be referred to. |
| **Targeted** | A decision regarding the patient most likely to benefit from a particular intervention. |
| **Timing** | A decision regarding the best time for an intervention. |

### Model for Ethical Decision Making

It is important for nurses to avoid making decisions solely based on their insistence that they know what is best for individuals. In 1998, Chally and Loriz developed the **Model for Ethical Decision Making** for nurses to use when faced with ethical dilemmas or choices. According to this model, steps to ethical decision making include the following:

1. Clarifying the extent/type of dilemma and who is ultimately responsible for making the decision.
2. Obtaining more data, including information about legal issues, such as the obligation to report.
3. Considering alternative solutions.
4. Arriving at a decision after considering risk/benefits and discussing it with the individual.
5. Acting on the decision and utilizing collaboration as needed.
6. Assessing the outcomes of the decision to determine if the chosen action was effective.

### Decision Making Tools and Techniques

#### *Brainstorming*

Brainstorming is a component of almost all planning and prioritizing activities. Brainstorming is used to generate ideas about problems, processes, solutions, or other criteria in a short time frame. Brainstorming may be structured, with each person in the group providing an idea in rotation, or unstructured, with people contributing at will. There are five primary steps:

1. Establish the purpose of the brainstorming and identify a time frame.
2. Decide between a structured vs. unstructured approach.
3. Allow time for general discussion or individual thought.

4. List ideas according to the approach. Ideas may be written on a white board or flip chart or projected from a computer so that the group can look at the list.
5. Discuss items, clarify them, and combine like items as the group agrees.

In some cases, members may be asked to rate or rank items on the list individually, and then points are assigned to each item and the list is prioritized accordingly. In some cases, other methods of prioritization may be used.

### *Multivoting*

Multivoting is a procedure used to prioritize and reach consensus when selecting process improvement activities. **Steps** include:

1. Review the initial list for redundancies/similarities and combine like items if the group agrees, restating the item as agreed by the team.
2. Number the remaining items on the list (without prioritizing).
3. Select a voting method, such as colored dots or a point system, or a ranking system. One method is one-half plus one (one dot more than half the number of items).
4. Vote—using whatever method was chosen—and then tally the votes to determine which items have the most votes.
5. Discuss top vote-getting items.
6. Eliminate items with no votes or few votes, and then vote again if necessary.
7. Repeat the revoting/discussing procedure until the list has narrowed, and then use the voting to prioritize the remaining items.

### *Affinity Diagram*

An affinity diagram is used to brainstorm and organize large numbers of ideas, items, or issues (>15) into major categories. **Steps** include:

1. Brainstorm to generate a list of ideas, with each one written on a sticky note or card.
2. Display the cards/sticky notes at random on a table or wall.
3. Sort cards/sticky notes into groups, silently and quickly, trying to find the first two ideas that go together, placing them to one side and then adding to that group until all cards have been either grouped or stand isolated. Discuss each group and agree for a title for each group. If some groups appear to be a subgroup, then subheadings may be created and one group moved as a subgroup under another.
4. Draw a diagram with the issue/problem at the top and then the major headings below that with lists beneath the headings.

## Leadership Styles

Leadership styles often influence the perception of leadership values and commitment to collaboration. There are a number of different **leadership styles**:

- **Charismatic:** Relies on personal charisma to influence people, and may be very persuasive, but this type leader may engage followers and relate to one group rather than the organization at large, limiting effectiveness.
- **Bureaucratic:** Follows organization rules exactly and expects everyone else to do so. This is most effective in handling cash flow or managing work in dangerous work environments. This type of leadership may engender respect but may not be conducive to change.

- **Autocratic:** Makes decisions independently and strictly enforces rules. Team members often feel left out of process and may not be supportive of the decisions that are made. This type of leadership is most effective in crisis situations, but may have difficulty gaining the commitment of staff.
- **Consultative:** Presents a decision and welcomes input and questions, although decisions rarely change. This type of leadership is most effective when gaining the support of staff is critical to the success of proposed changes.
- **Participatory:** Presents a potential decision and then makes final decision based on input from staff or teams. This type of leadership is time-consuming and may result in compromises that are not entirely satisfactory to management or staff, but this process is motivating to staff who feel their expertise is valued.
- **Democratic:** Presents a problem and asks staff or teams to arrive at a solution, although the leader usually makes the final decision. This type of leadership may delay decision-making, but staff and teams are often more committed to the solutions because of their input.
- **Laissez-faire ("Free Reign"):** Exerts little direct control but allows employees/teams to make decisions with little interference. This may be effective leadership if teams are highly skilled and motivated, but in many cases, this type of leadership is the product of poor management skills and little is accomplished because of this lack of leadership.

## SHARED GOVERNANCE

Shared governance implies shared decision making, but this can be realized in different ways. A common form of shared governance is for the administration to allow autonomous decision making by specific departments, teams, or groups within an organization regarding issues that apply to them or are within their area of expertise. For example, a unit team may have the authority to establish work schedules for that unit only, and members of a professional development team may be able to make decisions regarding professional development activities. In some cases, shared governance committees communicate with administration and can affect decision making but do not make the final decision. Members of shared governance teams or groups may be tasked with specific duties, such as developing new policies or procedures related to evidence-based best practices. Shared governance has primarily involved nursing personnel in most organizations.

### *PARTNERSHIP COUNCILS*

Partnership councils represent an evolution of shared governance, which focuses primarily on nursing. Partnership councils have members from all levels and areas within an organization. Thus, a partnership council may include all disciplines, such as nursing, laboratory, and housekeeping, and all departments. Partnership councils usually exist at different levels in an organization, so there may be department or unit partnership councils as well as a central partnership council that serves as an advisory board and shares decision making with the administration. Usually one member (most often a chairperson) of each unit or department partnership council becomes a representative on the central council so that communication moves both horizontally and vertically. This type of sharing of information and ideas helps to promote decision making that considers the system needs as well as the unit needs.

## SYSTEMS THEORY

Systems theory, developed by Ludwig von Bertalanffy in the 1940s, is an approach that considers the entire system holistically rather than focusing on component parts. Bertalanffy believed that all of the elements of a system and their interrelations needed to be understood because all interact in order to achieve goals, and change in any one element will impact the other elements, therefore alter outcomes. According to the systems theory, there are **four elements in a system**:

- **Input**: This is what goes into a system in terms of energy or materials.
- **Processes**: These are the actions that take place in order to transform input.
- **Output**: This is the result of the interrelationship between input and processes.
- **Feedback**: This is information that results and can be used for evaluation of the system.

To achieve desired outcomes, every part of the process must be considered. The individual parts added together do not constitute the whole because viewing the parts separately does not account for the dynamic quality of interaction that takes place.

### Neuman's Total-Person Systems Model

Betty Neuman developed the Total-Person Systems Model of nursing in 1972, which was inspired by the system theory. This model applies to the nursing professional development specialist. The concentric circle of variables (physiological, psychological, sociocultural, spiritual, and developmental) provides defense for the individual and should be considered simultaneously for the individual, who directly interacts with and is influenced by the environment. This model focuses on how the individual reacts to stress through mechanisms of defense and resistance and how this feedback affects that individual's stability. Stressors are environmental forces that may provide negative or positive reactions, affecting the individual's stability. Stressors may be intrapersonal, interpersonal, or extrapersonal. The nurse intervenes to help the individual maintain stability and prevent negative effects. Interventions include:

- **Primary** (health promotion, education): Preventive steps are taken prior to reaction to stressor.
- **Secondary**: Goal is to prevent damage of the central core by facilitating internal resistance and by removal of stressor.
- **Tertiary**: Efforts are made to promote reconstitution and reduce energy needs, supporting the client after secondary interventions.

## Organizational Principles and Concepts

### Organizational Culture

Organizational culture is very difficult to define, as it comprises the attitudes, beliefs, and behaviors of those involved in the organization. The physical environment and the organizational structure also impact culture. Culture involves shared assumptions about behavior and working together in an organization. Facilitating change within an organization must include understanding the basic underlying values and changing the organizational culture as well as changing processes and procedures. There are different **types of organizational cultures**:

- **Stable learning cultures** where people exercise skills and advance over time.
- **Independent cultures** in which people have valued skills that are easily transferable to other organizations.
- **Group cultures** in which there is strong identification and emphasis on seniority.
- **Insecure cultures** with frequent staff layoffs and reorganization.

Facilitating changes in the organizational culture requires a commitment to excellence at all levels with opportunities for involvement and empowerment of staff. Management must be flexible, encouraging team building and systems thinking across the organization.

## ORGANIZATIONAL DYNAMICS

An organization comprises two or more individual or subsystems that must work together to achieve outcomes that cannot be achieved in isolation. Organizational dynamics refer to the manner and effectiveness in which the individuals or subsystems work together. Homeostasis is a state of balance that an organization strives for through exchange of information, energy, and materials. The dynamic quality of organizations is such that any change in one component of a system has an effect on other components because none are able to function in isolation. Thus, when an organization is not functioning effectively, identifying the component or components that are having a negative effect is critical to quality improvement. However, identifying the component or components that are having a positive effect is equally important, as these components may serve as models for the rest of the organization.

## MISSION STATEMENT

The mission statement of an organization usually reflects the current status of the organization and describes, in broad terms, the purpose of the organization and its role in the community. The mission statement should be developed in response to data and program analysis and with input from all members of the organization. The mission statement should identify the organization or program, state its function, and outline the purpose and strategy of the program:

*The mission of Hospital X, a collaborative group of professionals, physicians, administrators, nurses, and support staff, is to promote health and safety of patients, visitors, and staff, and to provide outstanding quality healthcare services to the community.*

The mission statement should in some way include a commitment to quality and patient care as well as the need to serve the community. In many cases, the mission statement is followed by detailed explanations that may include statements of organizational values, philosophy, and history.

## VISION STATEMENT

An organizational vision statement requires analysis of both internal and external customer-supplier relationships in arriving at a statement about what the organization intends to become. The vision statement is the commitment that the organization is making. The vision statement should include future goals rather than focusing on what has already been achieved. The vision statement is usually stated in one sentence or a short paragraph:

*Hospital X will be the leader in providing sustainable quality patient-centered care to the community to improve the physical and mental health of community members.*

The vision statement is often followed by an explanation of terms, so that such concepts as "sustainable" and "patient-centered" are clarified to explain the reason for including the terms in the vision statement. For example, if "sustainable" is part of the vision statement, then the explanation may include the need to function within budget constraints while providing optimum care.

## ORGANIZATIONAL VALUES, GOALS, AND OBJECTIVES

The development of goals and objectives is done in support of the mission and vision statements and **organizational values** and should be completed at the same time to determine if the mission and vision statements can be realized and to explain how that will happen. **Goals** should be achievable aims, essentially end results, developed for specific units of the organization or the organization in general, focusing on improving performance. One example of a specific goal includes:

*Reduction in surgical site infections by 30%.*

In healthcare quality management, the goals must be based on knowledge about functions and processes within the organization and prioritized accordingly as part of achieving positive patient outcomes. **Objectives** are the measurable steps taken to achieve goals, and in the case of infections, an objective might include:

*An infection control professional will audit antibiotic use, and the physician internal medicine committee will establish antibiotic prophylaxis protocol within 6 months.*

Objectives should be measurable and should include a timeline and identification of responsibility for achieving the objective.

## Organizational Strategic Plan

Organization-wide strategic planning requires that an organization look at needs of the organization, community, and customers, and establish goals for not only the near future (2-4 years) but into the extended future (10-15 years). Strategic planning must be based on assessments, both internal and external, to determine the present courses of action, needed changes, priorities, and methodologies to effect change. The focus of strategic planning must be on development of services based on identified customer needs and then the marketing of those services. Organization-wide strategic planning includes:

- Collecting data and doing an external analysis of customer needs in relation to regulations and demographics.
- Analyzing internal services and functions.
- Identifying and understanding key issues, including the strengths and weaknesses of the organization as well as potential opportunities and negative impacts.
- Developing revised mission and vision statement that identifies core values.
- Establishing specific goals and objectives.

## Organizational Structure

### *Organizational Chart and Committee Structure*

An **organizational chart** is a diagram that shows the structure of an organization, indicating the relationship of one unit or department to another and showing the chain of command. The three most common types of organizational charts are hierarchical with the position of power at the top and those below in descending order. In the matrix format, management may be listed at the top but then each different department or unit listed on an equal basis. The horizontal format is similar to the matrix but the chain of command is very limited and department managers are fairly autonomous.

**Committee structure** varies from one organization to another but typically includes an executive committee and a number of subcommittees with responsibility for projects, departments, or concerns. Ad hoc committees are temporary committees formed to carry out a specific project or task, as opposed to standing committees, which are permanent.

### *Organizational Affiliations/Alignment*

Organizational or institutional **affiliations** are formal agreements between organizations or other entities. In an affiliation, organization A usually has the power to control organization B because of acquisition or contract, but organization B may be fairly autonomous. For example, a Catholic hospital may acquire a Jewish hospital but both hospitals may maintain their separate identities while sharing some resources and management. Organizational **alignment** usually refers to physician-organization alignment, which is coordination between the organization and the physician to better ensure compensation for services. Physician-organization alignment can be carried out in three different manners:

- **Independent physician**: A contractual arrangements formalizes services provided to physicians or by physicians who are autonomous.
- **Employed physician**: The organization acquires private practices or hires physicians directly, but this option is expensive.
- **Integrated network/accountable care organizations**: A formal program integrates the services of both independent physicians and employed physicians.

# Change Management

## Complex Adaptive Theory

According to the Complex Adaptive Theory, complex systems are interdisciplinary systems with multiple components or agents that depend on interaction and adaptation as part of learning. Adaptive systems are open systems that are able to adapt readily to changes and problems. The original adaptive theory referred to biology, but the model has expanded to encompass families, communities, and organizations. Interactions tend to be rich and nonlinear with close associates and with much feedback. Interactions are often random rather than planned. Change is often mutual: Agents change causing the system to change, and the system changes cause agents to change. Adaptive systems are dynamic by nature with interdependent agents acting together to bring about change. Adaptive systems that are self-adjusting are able to avoid chaos even though changes may bring them to the brink. Adaptive systems tend to favor effectiveness over efficiency and are less rule-governed than nonadaptive systems.

## Transtheoretical Model

The transtheoretical model focuses on changes in behavior based on the individual's decisions (not on society's decisions or others' decisions) and is used to develop strategies to promote changes in health behavior. This model outlines stages people go through when changing problem behavior and trying to have a positive attitude about change. **Stages of change** include the following:

- **Precontemplation**: The person is either unaware or under-informed about consequences of a problem behavior and has no intention of changing behavior within the next 6 months.
- **Contemplation**: The person is aware of costs and benefits of changing behavior and intends to change within the next 6 months but is procrastinating and not ready for action.
- **Preparation**: The person has a plan and intends to initiate change in the near future (≤1 month) and is ready for action plans.
- **Action**: The person is modifying behavior change occurs only if behavior meets a set criterion (such as complete abstinence from drinking).
- **Maintenance**: The person works to maintain changes and gains confidence that he or she will not relapse.

## Health Belief Model

The Health Belief Model (HBM), developed by Irwin Rosenstock (1966), is a model used to predict health behavior with the understanding that people take a health action to avoid negative consequences if the person expects that the negative outcome can be avoided and that he or she is able to do the action. The HBM, as modified, is based on six basic perceptions:

- **Susceptibility**: Belief that the person may get a negative condition.
- **Severity**: Understanding of how serious a condition is.
- **Benefit**: Belief that the action will reduce risk of getting the condition.
- **Barriers**: Direct and psychological costs involved in taking action.
- **Action cues**: Strategies used to encourage action, such as education.
- **Self-efficacy**: Confidence in the ability to take action and achieve positive results.

This model attempts to encourage people to make changes or take action (such as stopping smoking) in order to avoid negative consequences, so when this model is used for education, the educator focuses on the negative consequences (such as quitting smoking to avoid cardiovascular and pulmonary disease).

## Bowen's Family Systems Theory

Bowen's Family Systems Theory suggests that one must look at the person in terms of his or her family unit because the members of a family have different roles and behavioral patterns, so a change in one person's behavior will affect the others in the family. According to this model, there are eight interrelated concepts:

- **Triangle theory**: Two people comprise a basic unit, but when conflict occurs, a third person is drawn into the unit for stability with the resulting dynamic of two supporting one or two opposing one. This, in turn, draws in other triangles.
- **Self-differentiation**: People vary in need for external approval.
- **Nuclear family patterns**: Patterns include marital conflict, one spouse dysfunctional, one or more children impaired, and emotional distance.
- **Projection within a family**: Problems (emotional) passed from parent to child.
- **Transmission (multigenerational)**: Small differences in transmission from parent to child.
- **Emotional isolation**: Reducing or eliminating family contact.
- **Sibling order**: Influence on behavior and development.
- **Emotional process (society)**: Results in regressive or progressive social movements.

## Theory of Planned Behavior

The Theory of Planned Behavior, by Ajzen, evolved from the Theory of Reasoned Action in 1985 when studies showed that behavioral intention does not necessarily result in action. The Theory of Planned Behavior is more successful in predicting behavior. To the basic concepts of attitudes, subjective norms, and behavioral intentions encompassed by the earlier theory, Ajzen added the concept of perceived behavioral control, which relates to the individual's attitudes about self-efficacy and outcomes. Ajzen's theory shows that beliefs are central:

- **Behavioral beliefs** lead to attitudes toward a behavior/action.
- **Normative beliefs** lead to subjective norms.
- **Control beliefs** lead to perceived behavioral control.

All of these beliefs interact to influence intention and action. Basically, this theory relates to the person's confidence, based on beliefs and social influence of others, that he or she can actually do an action and that the outcome of this action will be positive. This theory looks at the power of emotions—such as apprehension or fear—when predicting behavior.

## Change Theory

Change Theory was developed by Kurt Lewin and modified by Edgar Schein. This management theory is based on three stages:

- Motivation to change (**unfreezing**): Dissatisfaction occurs when goals are not met, but as previous beliefs are brought into question, survival anxiety occurs, but sometimes learning anxiety about having to learn different strategies causes resistance that can lead to denial, blaming others, and trying to maneuver or bargain without real change.
- Desire to change (**unfrozen):** Dissatisfaction is strong enough to override defensive actions and the desire to change is strong, but must be coupled with identification of needed changes.
- Development of permanent change (**refreezing**): The new behavior that has developed becomes habitual, often requiring a change in perceptions of self and establishment of new relationships.

### *Force-Field Analysis*

Force field analysis was part of Kurt Lewin's Change Theory, meant to analyze both the driving forces and the restraining forces for change:

- **Driving forces** instigate and promote change, such as leaders, incentives, and competition.
- **Restraining forces** resist change, such as poor attitudes, hostility, inadequate equipment, or insufficient funds.

The professional development nurse can use this force field analysis diagram to discuss variables related to a proposed change in process:

- Write the proposed change in the center column.
- Brainstorm and list driving forces and opposed restraining forces. Score the forces. (When driving and restraining forces are in balance, this is a state of equilibrium or the status quo.)
- Discuss the value of the proposed change.
- Develop a plan to diminish or eliminate restraining forces.

## Facilitating Practice Change

Leadership within an organization must be consistent, and it succeeds by providing staff with direction and guidance that show by example, explaining why things need to be done rather than directing how this must be achieved. A good leader fosters **practice change** by focusing on the right way to do things rather than on errors or poor performance. By engaging staff in all part of the processes, a leader engenders a sense of commitment and collaboration on the part of the staff. This commitment cannot be achieved through rules, regulation, threats, and criticism. A good leader must demonstrate integrity, welcome diversity, be open-minded, and search for competence. While a leader must have a thorough understanding of the organization/facility and its work, he or she must be able to observe holistically. The leader must motivate others by providing structure, order, and the ability to make decisions while continuing to learn and teach in order to create positive change.

# Communication Principles and Methods

## CHARACTERISTICS OF COMMUNICATION

Characteristics of communication include:

- **Process**: Communication is a complex dynamic process that is bidirectional and involves both verbal and nonverbal interactions.
- **Symbolic**: Communication always uses symbols of some type to transmit thoughts and ideas. Almost anything can become a symbol to transmit information: images, words, appearance, color, tone of voice. The same symbol may transmit something very different to different receivers, who translate the symbol received into meaning.
- **Receiver-based**: Communication occurs with the receiver when meaning is attached to symbol. All behavior communicates whether intended or not.
- **Irreversible**: Once communication occurs, it cannot be withdrawn or reversed. Correction of unintended communication may communicate a different message but the original remains.
- **Unrepeatable**: An original communication can never be repeated in the exact same way because the communication process is dependent on the receiver.

## RECIPIENT CHARACTERISTICS

Communication is dependent on the recipient of the intended or unintended message because the transfer of information is affected by recipient's motivation to decode the message and ability to comprehend the message. If a recipient lacks motivation, then communication as intended may be effectively blocked or a completely different message received. For example, if the recipient does not want to hear a message and pays no attention to the actual content, the message received may be that the communicator is annoying or overbearing. Therefore, for effective communication to occur, the recipient must be motivated to receive the message. The ability of the recipient to comprehend a message depends on many complex factors, such as cognitive ability, knowledge base, emotional status, sensory impairment, and health status. For example, if a person is hard of hearing, a spoken message may be incomprehensible.

## THERAPEUTIC COMMUNICATION

Therapeutic communication begins with respect for the patient/family/staff member and the assumption that all communication, verbal and nonverbal, has meaning. Listening must be done empathetically. The following are some techniques that facilitate communication.

**Introduction**:

- Make a personal introduction and use the patient's name: "Mrs. Brown, I am Susan Williams, your nurse."

**Encouragement**:

- Use an open-ended opening statement: "Is there anything you'd like to discuss?"
- Acknowledge comments: "Yes," and "I understand."
- Allow silence and observe nonverbal behavior rather than trying to force conversation. Ask for clarification if statements are unclear.
- Reflect statements back (use sparingly): Patient: "I hate this hospital." Nurse: "You hate this hospital?"

**Empathy:**

- Make observations: "You are shaking," and "You seem worried."
- Recognize feelings:
    - Patient: "I want to go home."
    - Nurse: "It must be hard to be away from your home and family."
- Provide information as honestly and completely as possible about condition, treatment, and procedures and respond to the patient's questions and concerns.

**Exploration:**

- Verbally express implied messages:
    - Patient: "This treatment is too much trouble."
    - Nurse: "You think the treatment isn't helping you?"
- Explore a topic but allow the patient to terminate the discussion without further probing: "I'd like to hear how you feel about that."

**Orientation:**

- Indicate reality:
    - Patient: "Someone is screaming."
    - Nurse: "That sound was an ambulance siren."
- Comment on distortions without directly agreeing or disagreeing:
    - Patient: "That nurse promised I didn't have to walk again."
    - Nurse: "Really? That's surprising because the doctor ordered physical therapy twice a day."

**Collaboration:**

- Work together to achieve better results: "Maybe if we talk about this, we can figure out a way to make the treatment easier for you."

**Validation:**

- Seek validation: "Do you feel better now?" or "Did the medication help you breathe better?"

## Nontherapeutic Communication

While using therapeutic communication is important, it is equally important to avoid interjecting non-therapeutic communication, which can block effective communication. **Avoid the following:**

- Meaningless clichés: "Don't worry. Everything will be fine." "Isn't it a nice day?"
- Providing advice: "You should..." or "The best thing to do is...." It's better when patients ask for advice to provide facts and encourage the patient to reach a decision.
- Inappropriate approval that prevents the patient from expressing true feeling or concerns:
    - Patient: "I shouldn't cry about this."
    - Nurse: "That's right! You're an adult!"
- Asking for an explanation of behavior that is not directly related to patient care and requires analysis and explanation of feelings: "Why are you so upset?"

- Agreeing with rather than accepting and responding to patient's statements can make it difficult for the patient to change his or her statement or opinion later: "I agree with you," or "You are right."
- Making negative judgments: "You should stop arguing with the nurses."
- Devaluing the patient's feelings: "Everyone gets upset at times."
- Disagreeing directly: "That can't be true," or "I think you are wrong."
- Defending against criticism: "The doctor is not being rude; he's just very busy today."
- Changing the subject to avoid dealing with uncomfortable topics;
    - Patient: "I'm never going to get well."
    - Nurse: "Your family will be here in just a few minutes."
- Making inappropriate literal responses, even as a joke, especially if the patient is at all confused or having difficulty expressing ideas:
    - Patient: "There are bugs crawling under my skin."
    - Nurse: "I'll get some bug spray,"
- Challenging the patient to establish reality often just increases confusion and frustration:
    - "If you were dying, you wouldn't be able to yell and kick!"

## Nonverbal Communication

Nonverbal communication can convey as much information as verbal communication, both on the nurse's part and the patient's. Nonverbal communication is used for a number of purposes, such as expressing feelings and attitudes, and may be a barrier to communication or a facilitator. While there are cultural differences, interpretation of nonverbal communication can help the nurse to better understand and promote communication:

- **Eye contact**: Making eye contact (within the American culture) provides a connection and shows caring and involvement in the communication. Avoiding contact may indicate someone is not telling the truth or is uncomfortable, fearful, ashamed, or hiding something.
- **Tone**: The manner in which words are spoken (patiently, cheerfully, somberly) affects the listener, and when the message and tone do not match, it can interfere with communication. A high-pitched tone of voice may indicate nervousness or stress.
- **Touch**: Reaching out to touch an older adult's hand or pat a shoulder during communication is reassuring but hugging or excessive touching can make people feel uncomfortable. People may touch themselves (lick lips, pick at skin, scratch) if they are anxious.
- **Gestures**: Using the hands to emphasize meaning is common and may be particularly helpful during explanations, but excessive gesturing can be distracting. Some gestures alone convey message, such as a wave goodbye or pointing. Tapping of the foot, moving the legs, or fidgeting may indicate nervousness. Rubbing the hands together is sometimes a self-comforting measure. Some gestures, such as handshakes, are part of social ritual. Mixed messages, such as fidgeting but speaking with a calm voice, may indicate uncertainty or anxiety.
- **Posture**: Slumping can indicate lack of interest or withdrawal. Leaning toward the opposite person while talking indicates interest and facilitates interaction.

## Passive Communication

Passive communication occurs when the individual does not express an opinion directly or verbally but may communicate in a non-direct or nonverbal manner. The passive communicator may be non-committal and submissive, often contributing little to a conversation and unwilling to take sides in a conflict. The person may believe that personal opinions are not important and may avoid direct eye contact and appear nervous and fidgety if confronted. The individual may show signs of anxiety, such as wringing hands and crossing the arms. The passive communicator may respond inappropriately when angry, such as by laughing, and may believe that disagreeing with another person will be upsetting to that person or result in conflict, which the communicator wants to avoid. The passive communicator benefits by rarely being blamed for failures (since the person took little part in decision making) and by avoiding conflict (at least short-term).

## Assertive Communication

Assertive communication occurs when the individual expresses opinions directly and actions correlate with words. Assertive communicators are respectful of others and not bullying but firm and honest about opinions. They frequently use "I" statements to make their point: "I would like...". Communication usually includes cooperative statements, such as "What do you think?" and distinguishes between fact and opinion. Assertive communicators often engender trust in others because they are consistent, honest, and open in communicating with others. The assertive communicator feels free to express disagreement and anger, but does so in a manner that is nonthreatening and respectful of others' feelings. Assertive communication requires a strong sense of self-worth and the belief that personal opinions have value. Assertive communicators tend to have good listening skills because they value the opinions of others and feel comfortable collaborating.

## Aggressive Communication

Aggressive communication has some of the same characteristics as assertive communication but lacks the respect for others. The aggressive communicator expresses opinions directly and forcefully but does not want to hear the opinions of others and may denigrate those who speak up or disagree. The aggressive communicator often bullies others into agreement but is usually disliked, and this can increase social anxiety and resentment, leading to further aggression. The aggressive communicator may use sarcasms or insults and may frequently interrupt or talk over other speakers and may intrude on others' personal space. They often believe they are superior to others or more intelligent and may take an aggressive stand (standing upright, feet apart, hands on hips). Hand gestures may include making fists and pointing fingers at others. Benefits of aggressive communication are being in control, getting one's own way, and feeling powerful.

## Cultural and Spiritual Competence

A number of issues are related to cultural and spiritual competence in communicating with patients/family, including the following:

- **Eye contact**: Many cultures use eye contact differently than is common in the United States. They may avoid direct eye contact, considering it rude, or may look away to signal disapproval, or may look down to signal respect. Careful observation of the way family members use eye contact can help to determine what will be most comfortable for the patient/family.
- **Distance**: Staff are not legally required to ask. There is considerable difference relating to concepts of personal space among cultures. Allowing the family to approach or observing whether they tend to move closer, lean forward, or move back can help to determine a comfortable distance for communication.
- **Time**: Americans tend to be time-oriented, and expect people to be on time, but time is more flexible in many cultures, so scheduling may require flexibility.

## Workplace Communication

### Charts and Graphs

Presenting data in the form of **charts and graphs** provides a visual representation of the data that is easy to comprehend, facilitating communication. There are basically three types of graphs:

- **Line graphs** have an x and y axis, so they are used to show how an independent variable affects a dependent variable. Line graphs can show a time series with time usually on the x (horizontal) axis. This graph might be used to show number of infections per week/month.
- **Bar graphs** are used to compare and show the relationship between two or more groups. The graphs can show quantifiable data as bars that extend horizontally, vertically, or stacked. Bar graphs might be used to show comparison data of different populations or to compare data from one time period to another.
- **Pie charts** are used to show what percentage an item is compared with the whole. A pie chart can show distribution of infection control resources.

### Flow Charts

A flow chart is a tool of quality improvement and is used to provide a pictorial/schematic representation of a process. It is a particularly helpful tool for communicating quality improvement projects when each step in a process is analyzed while searching for solutions to a problem. Typically, the following symbols are used:

- **Parallelogram**: Input and output (start/end)
- **Arrow**: Direction of flow
- **Diamond-shape**: Conditional decision (yes/no or true/false)
- **Circles**: Connectors with diverging paths with multiple arrows coming in but only one going out.

A variety of other symbols may be used as well to indicate different functions. Flow goes from top to bottom and left to right. Flow charts are particularly helpful for visualizing how a process is carried out and examining a process for problems. Flow charts may also be used to plan a process before it is utilized. Flow charts may also be used to demonstrate critical pathways to outline treatment options/paths related to findings.

### Barriers

Barriers to effective workplace communication include:

- **Psychological factors**: The communicator's or recipient's emotional status, such as increased anxiety, can negatively impact communication. Biases, prejudices, and belief systems may also interfere with a person's ability to attend to the ideas of another person.
- **Physical factors**: Communication may be impaired if there is excessive noise or distracting activities taking place. Some environments are not conducive to communication, especially if too great a distance separates communicators.
- **Gender factors**: Communication styles often vary between males and females, and this can lead to misunderstanding. However, communication styles may also vary among those of the same gender, depending on many social and psychological factors.
- **Semantic factors**: Communicators may have different understanding of the same words. For example, a speaker of English as a second language may have a more literal interpretation of words than a native speaker, and this can lead to misunderstanding.

## INTERPERSONAL COMMUNICATION SKILLS

Collaboration requires a number of communication skills that differ from those involved in communication between nurse and patient. These skills include:

- **Using an assertive approach:** It's important for the nurse to honestly express opinions and to state them clearly and with confidence, but the nurse must do so in a calm, non-threatening manner.
- **Making casual conversation:** It's easier to communicate with people with whom one has a personal connection. Asking open-ended questions, asking about other's work, or commenting on someone's contributions helps to establish a relationship. The time before meetings, during breaks, and after meetings presents an opportunity for this type of conversation.
- **Being competent in public speaking:** Collaboration requires that a nurse be comfortable speaking and presenting ideas to groups of people. Speaking and presenting ideas competently also helps the nurse to gain credibility. Public speaking is a skill that must be practiced.
- **Communicating in writing:** The written word remains a critical component of communication, and the nurse should be able to communicate clearly and grammatically.

### *SENDER-RECEIVER FEEDBACK LOOP*

The communication process, which includes the sender-receiver feedback loop, is based on Claude Shannon's information theory (1948) in which he described three necessary steps: encoding a message, transmitting through a channel, and decoding. The resultant communication process begins with the sender, who serves as the encoder and determines the content of the message. The medium is the form the message takes (digital, written, audiovisual), and the channel is the method of delivery (mail, radio, TV, phone). The recipient (receiver) who acts as the decoder determines the meaning from the message. Feedback helps to determine whether or not the communication was successful and the message was understood as intended. This process is referred to as the send-receiver feedback loop. Context is the environment (physical and psychological) in which the communication occurs, and interference is any factor that impacts the communication process. Interference may be external (such as environmental noise) or internal (such as emotional distress or anxiety).

## COMMUNICATION IN RELATION TO CUSTOMER SERVICE

Customer service involves interpersonal communication with a customer to attend to the person's needs. This communication may be face-to-face or via telephone, email, internet chat, or text messaging. For face-to-face and telephone communication, the customer service individual must have strong verbal communication skills. For email, internet chat, or text messaging, the individual must also have good typing and grammar skills. The customer service individual should be knowledgeable about the needs of customers, have up-to-date information, and understand the level of authority needed to respond to customers' needs. In all cases, the individual must exhibit patience and have a good understanding of behavioral psychology in order to assess the customer's emotional status. It is important for the individual to listen attentively to customers and to use positive language in response. The individual must also have good time management skills in order to avoid wasting time with customers.

## NEED TO KNOW AS IT RELATES TO NURSE-PATIENT COMMUNICATION

Patients have a right to expect that when they divulge personal information to a nurse that only those with a need to know (such as the physician and other nurses) will be provided this information. When nurses must document care, they must be sensitive to the information that they put into the written record or report because many people have access to these records. If the information is health related, then the nurse is obligated to record this and should tell the patient. Need to know issues also relate to the patient's need to know about care and prognosis. Patients may be overwhelmed by information or, if they are cognitively impaired, confused. Older adults and families should be asked how much information they want. Some patients/families want to know all of the details, including treatment options and expected outcomes. Others want only the basic information or do not want to discuss health issues at all.

### INFORMATION SHARING/NETWORKING

A number of different computers in different locations can be linked together by networking software to facilitate information sharing. Networks also may allow for sharing of resources, such as all computers in a room using the same printer. Networks may be used to facilitate telenursing and e-health programs, research, and educational programs. Virtual social networks allow participants to share information and expertise. Different **types of networks** include:

- **Local-area network (LAN):** Computers in the network are in a relatively small area, such as one room or one building. An intranet is a type of LAN that serves the role of a secure private internet. An extranet allows suppliers or other business partners to connect to each other's network.
- **Wide-area network (WAN):** This allows computers to connect over large distances, such as a state, a country, or the entire world. The internet is a prime example of a WAN.

### SELECTING APPROPRIATE COMMUNICATION METHODS

Selecting appropriate communication methods requires a number of steps:

1. Consider the purpose of the communication.
2. Identify the person(s) that will be the recipients and obtain or consider information about them, what influences them, and how best to reach them.
3. Consider the message to be conveyed and the best way to communicate so that the message is received as intended.
4. Determine whether the communication is intended as one-way or requires feedback. Choose an interactive channel if feedback is desired.
5. Determine the cost or effort involved in communicating through the chosen channel.
6. Develop the correct format for the communication (letter, fax, email), using or developing a template as appropriate.
7. Complete the message and carry out the communication using the channel selected.
8. Monitor feedback if appropriate.

#### *WRITTEN COMMUNICATION*

Written communication includes a wide range of choices in which the written word can be utilized. Written communication is most often used for formal proposals, advertisements, brochures, and letters. Contracts are almost always completed in hardcopy written form. However, email messages and documents are now often taking the place of hardcopy written documents because of less cost and more rapid communication. When utilizing written communication, the writer must consider the purpose of the communication and the structure of the document and the style in which is it written. Templates may be used for structure, but style and content depend on the writer. The information should be well organized with key points clearly outlined and supporting facts included. The introduction should create interest and the conclusion should provide a summary or suggestion for the future. The style of the writing should be appropriate for the recipient and may range from very formal to very informal. Paragraphs should be short, especially for online communications.

### *Verbal/Spoken Communication*

Verbal (spoken) communication can vary from very formal (such as a conference presentation) to very informal (such as a chat with a friend), but every aspect of the communication process has meaning—the words, the posture, the tone of voice, the expression on the face, silence times, and the general appearance. The communication of the same words will be very different if heard over the phone, read in an email, or heard face-to-face. In any professional communication, formal or informal, the individual should come prepared and should have some idea of what to say, although memorizing word-for-word is not advisable because communication should appear spontaneous even when it is not. The average person speaks about 200 words per minute and each sentence is a new creation; therefore, without planning, the message can easily become muddled. For formal presentation, brief outline notes or presentation software may be helpful to keep focused on the topic.

## Matching Communication Needs with Communication Vehicles

### *Mail, Email, Telephone, and Smartphone*

The **communication vehicle** utilized should best meet the communication needs:

- **Mail**: Use to add a personal touch to messages and to deliver documents securely. Mailings can reach large populations but cost may be relatively high.
- **Email**: Allows for fast communication and mass mailings at little cost, but emails are often screened and may be ignored if the receiver does not know or recognize the sender. Documents can be easily transmitted through email as text or PDF files.
- **Telephones (Landlines):** Use when interaction and discussion is needed or for personal appeals. The system should include voice mail. This is a relatively inexpensive form of communication, but the ubiquitous use of voice mail often means delays in actual communication.
- **Smartphones**: Use when rapid communication by phone, email, or messaging is needed as well as internet access. This is especially useful when the person is mobile.

### *Video/Web Conferencing, Internet/Webpages, Social Media, and Fax*

- **Video/Web conferencing**: This is valuable when participants cannot otherwise meet face to face and can save money associated with travel expenses. This vehicle allows participants to communicate both verbally and nonverbally.
- **Internet/Webpages**: Internet communication can be synchronous or asynchronous and allows for the presentation of information (such as on a webpage) as well as verbal communication (such as with messaging).
- **Social media**: These provide the opportunity to share professional or organizational information (such as with LinkedIn and Facebook). Twitter may be used to communicate short messages, and the messages should contain hashtags so interest can be assessed.
- **Fax**: This allows transfer of documents or images quickly and may be used, for example, to send an agenda prior to a meeting or to send documents that must be reviewed. Almost any type of document can be scanned and faxed.

#### Communications with Social Media

Social media include such sites as Facebook, LinkedIn, Twitter, and SnapChat. Social media are increasingly utilized for marketing, especially to younger generations who grew up with computers and the internet. Content developed for social media should be highly focused and of good quality if it is to attract an audience. Taking the time to identify and target influential individuals is an essential strategy in marketing because they can share content and expand outreach, at no additional cost, over social media. Personal communication via social media is more problematic because of the possibility of transmitting confidential or damaging information. Some organizations now prohibit their employees from making any mention of their organization in any social media, so any comments about employment or pictures must be avoided, whether positive or negative. One should never communicate negatively about an employer or anyone else on any social media site with an expectation of privacy and should avoid all comments that may be construed as racist, misogynistic, or bigoted.

### SCRIPTING

Scripting (a prewritten message) is a method used to ensure that communication is consistent among different individuals, such as when staff members are orienting patients. When creating a script, the first step is to determine the purpose and the message the script should convey. Generally, the first words of the script will focus on the topic and the purpose, "Mrs. Smith, we need to review your preparation for the colonoscopy." The script may explain the value to the individual and end with a summary. Scripts are particularly helpful for telephone triage or when responding to customer service requests. In most cases, the script should serve as a guideline rather than a narrative that should be memorized and recited verbatim or read; script users should practice and engage in roleplaying in order to become adept at staying on script as much as possible.

## Collaboration and Negotiation

### INTERDISCIPLINARY COLLABORATION

Interdisciplinary collaboration is absolutely critical to nursing practice if the needs and best interests of the individuals and families are central. Interdisciplinary practice begins with the nurse and physician but extends to pharmacists, social workers, occupational and physical therapists, nutritionists, and a wide range of allied healthcare providers, all of whom cooperate in diagnosis and treatment, but state regulations determine to some degree how much autonomy a nurse can have in diagnosing and treating. While nurses have increasingly gained more legal rights, they have also become more dependent upon collaboration with others for their expertise and for referrals if the individual's needs extend beyond the nurse's ability to provide assistance. Additionally, the prescriptive ability of advanced practice nurses varies from state to state, with some requiring direct supervision by other disciplines (such as physicians) while others require particular types of supervisory arrangements, depending upon the circumstances.

### PROMOTING COLLABORATION

Promoting collaboration and assisting others to understand and use resources and expertise of others require a commitment in terms of time and effort:

- Coaching others on methods of collaboration can include providing information in the form of handouts about effective communication strategies and, in turn, modeling this type of communication with the staff being coached.
- Team meetings are commonly held on nursing units, and they provide an opportunity to model collaboration and suggest the need for outside expertise to help with patient care plans. The mentoring nurse can initiate discussions about resources that are available in the facility or the community.

- Selecting a diverse group for teams or inviting those with expertise in various areas to join the team when needed can help team members to appreciate and understand how to use the input of other resources.

## Internal and External Collaboration

Collaboration through interdisciplinary teams is very common in health care and is a form of **internal collaboration** intended to improve health care. Internal collaboration takes place within an organization or program and may be formal or informal. A typical form of collaboration occurs when, for example, a nurse discusses how best to meet a patient's needs with an occupational therapist, benefitting from the knowledge of another professional. Internal collaboration is often face-to-face but may also be carried out by phone, text message, or email, especially in large organizations where opportunities for face-to-face meetings are limited.

**External collaboration** is often more formal and involves collaboration with those outside the organization often brought about by alliances, partnerships, and joint ventures. External collaboration may be motivated by the need for expertise not available in-house. External collaboration may be facilitated by technology, such as video-voice conferencing.

## Levels of Collaboration

Levels of collaboration include:

- **Nursing**: Individual nurses at all levels of the profession are in unique positions to ask questions about current practice and to work together to utilize evidence in practice, serving as role models and facilitating system-wide change.
- **Organizational**: Healthcare organizations respond to accreditation agencies and insurance companies as well as professional and governmental organizations and agencies in the development of changes in patient care based on research.
- **Regional**: Healthcare organizations, educational programs, libraries, and research programs, often cooperate in meeting healthcare needs in a region, such as a county, state, or regions of the country.
- **National**: Governmental agencies, such as AHRQ and the CDC, and professional organizations, such as the ANA and AMA, have been instrumental in providing guidance to healthcare organizations and promoting change.
- **International**: International organizations, such as the Cochrane Collaboration and World Health Organization (WHO), ensure that health information is available worldwide.

## Presentation of Evidence During Collaboration and Negotiation

The presentation of evidence is an important element of collaboration and negotiation. The presentation should be tailored to the audience, using appropriate language, and the discussion should include:

- **Overview**: An explanation of the type of research and evidence, the outcomes, and the potential for integrating the results of this research into current practice.
- **Validity**: A discussion of the manner in which the research was conducted, the type of research format, and explanation of how the research exhibits external validity.
- **Reliability**: The outcomes of the research should be completely explored, including effectiveness and any problems encountered.
- **Applicability**: The possible benefits to applying the research to practice must be clearly outlined, including discussion of how the research population aligns with the target population as well as how feasible (and cost-effective) implementation would be.

## APPROACHES TO NEGOTIATION

**Negotiating** may be a formal process (such as negotiating with administration for increased benefits) or informal process (such as arriving at a team consensus), depending on the purpose and those involved. Approaches to negotiation vary, including the following:

| | |
|---|---|
| **Competition** | In this approach, one party wins and the other loses, such as when parties feel their positions are nonnegotiable and are unwilling to compromise. To prevail, one party must remain firm, but this can result in conflict. |
| **Accommodation** | One party concedes to the other, but the losing side may gain little or nothing, so this approach should be used when there is clear benefit to one choice. |
| **Avoidance** | When both parties dislike conflict, they may put off negotiating and resolve nothing, so that the problems remain. |
| **Compromise** | Both parties make concessions in order to reach consensus, but this can result in decisions that suit no one, so compromise is not always the ideal solution. |
| **Collaboration** | Both parties receive what they want, often through creative solutions, but collaboration may be ineffective with highly competitive parties. |

## CONSULTATION

The nursing professional development specialist should develop and follow a consistent pattern of steps in consultation, understanding that each situation is distinct and may require flexibility. Usual **steps** include:

1. **Assessment**: The consultant must first assess the appropriateness of the request for consultation and the nature of the request, determining whether it is client centered, consultant centered, or program centered. The consultant must obtain data in order to identify the exact nature of the problem.
2. **Recommendations**: Based on data and observation, the consultant recommends interventions, such as further education or training for the consultee, clinical recommendations, or changes in processes.
3. **Documentation**: The consultant documents findings and recommendations and establishes a method of evaluation (survey, data, observation, outcomes).
4. **Evaluation**: The consultant uses appropriate feedback from evaluation to determine the effectiveness of the consultation.

### *PRINCIPLES OF CONSULTATION*

A number of principles of consultation have resulted from consultation theory:

- The consultee initiates the consultation in order to meet specific needs.
- The consultant and consultee operate in a horizontal rather than vertical relationship and collaborate to reach solutions to problems.
- The consultant looks at problems and challenges in context rather than in isolation.
- The consultant does not assume responsibility for management of patient care and does not have direct authority.
- The consultant makes recommendations only. Recommendations should be presented in an objective, nonjudgmental manner.

- The consultee is not under obligation to follow the recommendations of the consultant. The consultee makes the decision as to whether to accept or reject the consultant's recommendations.
- Consultation must be well documented, explaining not only the recommendations but also the observations and rationale for the recommendations.

### *Internal and External Consultation*

**Internal consulting** occurs within an institution or facility by a consultant who is a direct employee. Advantages to internal consultants include cost-effectiveness, especially if consultation is needed on an ongoing basis; familiarity with goals, mission, and needs of institution; ability to respond quickly; and maintenance of institutional privacy. However, internal consultants may have bias and may not represent best practices.

**External consulting** occurs when a consultant is contracted for a particular purpose, based on expertise. Advantages include the ability to find an expert in a specific area and cost-effectiveness if consultation is needed for only a prescribed period of time. The hourly wage may be higher but benefit costs are lower. Additionally, the contract can more easily be terminated if results are unsatisfactory. Disadvantages include less control over institutional privacy, increased time needed for the consultant to become familiar with the institution, and less commitment to the institution's goals.

### *Contracting, Engaging, and Disengaging*

Contracting for consultation services may be a formal or informal process in which temporary services are acquired for provision of staff augmentation or expertise. Informal consultation often occurs internally. External consultation is usually more formal. The consultation process involves contracting, engaging, and disengaging:

1. **Contracting** involves a formal contract that should outline the expected services, including outcomes and/or products, and should include the duration of services as well as any remuneration.
2. **Engaging** is the process of implementing the contract. During this stage, objectives and methods are outlined and the work plan developed as the consultant determines how to best meet the terms of the contract. Engaging also refers to the process by which the consultant and others develop a vested interest in the organization and the project.
3. **Disengaging** is the stage in which the consultant completes the contract and ends the consultative process. This may be planned (such as a time-limited contract), based on completion of a project, or requested by any party to the agreement.

## Situational Awareness and Environmental Scanning

### Searching for and Identifying Current and Future Trends

The professional development nurse should monitor key trends in nursing, health care, and other disciplines, and incorporate them into educational programs and activities. Key trends may be identified through literature review, observation, newsletters, continuing education, medical news, and conference attendance. **Key trends across the disciplines** include:

- Use of miniaturized or portable medical devices and robotic-assisted surgical devices.
- Social networking, internet access and research, and need for IT specialists.
- Nursing involvement in information technology and systems analysis.
- Utilization of home health care and decreased length of hospital stay.

- Focus on wellness, nutrition, preventive care, sustainability, and recycling.
- Individualized patient care.
- Flexible working hours and cost-containment methods.
- Specialization, certification, and interprofessional education.
- Gender, racial, and ethnic diversity among staff and patients.
- Focus on teamwork and interdisciplinary teams, patient satisfaction, and patient outcomes.

# Resource Management

## Competency Management Process

### *Clinical Competence*

Clinical competence is a primary concern of leadership, and expectations about competency should be clearly outlined during orientation to a position, including a complete job description that explains duties and expected skill level. A commonly used competency management process is for the individual to utilize a checklist of necessary basic skills and safety measures with performance assessed by peers or supervisors. If an individual lacks competence in some area, then a plan for remediation, training, or education to master the necessary skills must be carried out. An action plan should be developed to clarify the steps the individual must take to improve competence and the timeline for doing so, as well as an explanation of the manner in which competence will be assessed and the consequences of failure. The action plan should include a signed learner contract in which the individual agrees to follow specific steps of remediation to ensure compliance.

### *Contract Employees and Travelers*

**Contract employees** are employed for a specified period of time, sometimes as short as 1 day. Generally, they are contracted through an employment agency when a hospital or healthcare organization is short-staffed. In some cases, a hospital may contract with an individual directly for a specific short-term or long-term project.

**Traveler workers** include nurses, physicians, and therapists. Travel nurse agencies have proliferated, and costs are usually higher than when hiring locally. Typically, a traveling nurse works under contract for a limited period of time, such as 4-12 weeks, although some assignments may last up to 2 years. Most agencies require 1-2 years nursing experience for hire. Nurses may have to relicense if moving to another state unless it is part of the Nurse Licensure Compact. The hospital pays the agency, which in turn pays the nurse, so the nurse is not an actual employee of the hospital and not eligible for benefits provided to direct employees.

## Resource Management

### *Teams and Projects*

Resource management for teams and projects includes:

- **Resource assignment**: This involves selecting team members for specific projects, ensuring the best fit for the needs of the project. Negotiation or incentives may be needed to convince individuals to join a team and work in a project. Procedures should be in place for hiring any contract workers that will be needed.
- **Resource loading**: This refers to the number of human resources that are required during a specific period of the schedule. Over-allocation means more than the available resources are assigned to perform tasks at specific times. For example, an individual may be assigned to four tasks simultaneously even though this is not possible.

- **Resource leveling**: This involves delaying noncritical tasks, often as a solution to over-allocation. This may be effective if there is designated slack time built into the schedule; however, it can result in a delay in completion time.

### *Staffing Costs and Overtime*

Staffing costs, especially overtime, is always costly to an employer, because the federal Fair Labor Standards Act (FLSA) requires that an employee who works more than 40 hours per week be paid 1.5 times his or her regular hourly wage. Therefore, authorizing overtime on a frequent basis may cost the organization more money than if it hires another PTE (part-time employee) or FTE (full-time equivalent). Regularly exceeding the staffing budget increases the likelihood of the manager receiving a poor performance appraisal. Overworked employees are more likely to be injured or produce errors and are often inefficient. To minimize overtime, the staff should be large enough to accommodate all of the organization's needs. On-call employees should be designated for unscheduled absences. Job descriptions, QA analyses, and time-motion studies can be used to accurately estimate task completion times and to properly schedule staff.

### *Prioritization Matrix*

A prioritization matrix is used to prioritize items or select one from a number of alternatives based on preselected criteria. It can be helpful in the process of resource management. There are a number of **steps** involved with utilization of a prioritization matrix:

1. Use a brainstorming technique to generate a list of problems or options.
2. Select a group of criteria, such as "cost," "patient outcomes," or "safety."
3. Determine the relative value of each criterion and assign weighted points accordingly. For example, each vote for safety may be worth 2 points and cost 1 point.
4. Create a table with about 5-6 columns (to fit the number of criteria).
5. The heading for the left column will be "Problems/Options," and for the right column, it will be "Total Points." The middle columns contain the criteria.
6. Team members vote using a preselected method: check marking those criteria that apply, using a 1-5 scale for least to most important, using a yes/no system or + and –.
7. Total the scores to determine priorities.

### *Record Management*

#### Hardcopy Records

Managing information in relation to hardcopy materials is relatively straightforward. Materials are stored in some type of file or storage container, usually organized alphabetically by name, date, or department (or some combination), and placed in a secure room or facility. Organization systems vary widely, and so does security, which may be only a locked door. To retrieve materials, some type of procedure must be in place to review or sign out material in storage, but this can also vary. In some facilities, people needing files must gain access to the storage area and search for materials themselves, resulting in the potential for a lack of security as they may remove files or access unauthorized material. In other facilities, an authorized person retrieves files and other materials for those requesting information. However, documents can easily be removed or altered and files or materials misfiled, especially if people are allowed to remove them from the storage area, so that retrieving information can become difficult.

#### Digital Records

Managing information in relation to digital materials can be quite complex. While individual departments can store records, storage capacity may be quickly reached. In some facilities, medical information from different departments, such as the laboratory and clinical units, are stored on separate servers, so retrieving information may be time-consuming and difficult. Raw data and reports must be saved and securely stored in such a way that access is limited to authorized personnel only because of regulations related to privacy and confidentiality. Digital recordings may be stored electronically with backup so that data are not lost. Digital files may vary in size from 50-150+ megabytes, which can usually be stored on the individual computer system, but eventually the files need to be archived to make room for other recordings. This may mean transferring the information to an external hard drive, a recordable device (CD or DVD), or an optical disc. Data may also be transferred to a large central database or cloud storage.

## Team Management

### *Leading Teams*

Leading, facilitating, and participating in performance improvement teams requires a thorough understanding of the dynamics of **team building:**

- **Initial interactions:** This is the time when members begin to define their roles and develop relationships, determining if they are comfortable in the group.
- **Power issues:** The members observe the leader and determine who controls the meeting and how control is exercised, beginning to form alliances.
- **Organizing:** Methods to achieve work are clarified and team members begin to work together, gaining respect for each other's contributions and working toward a common goal.
- **Team identification:** Interactions often become less formal as members develop rapport, and members are more willing to help and support each other to achieve goals.
- **Excellence:** This develops through a combination of good leadership, committed team members, clear goals, high standards, external recognition, spirit of collaboration, and a shared commitment to the process.

### *Team Contracts*

Many of the problems that arise in team processes could be avoided if the team members reached consensus about expectations of working within the group. One method of team building is to complete a **team contract** at an initial meeting with all members participating. Team contracts should include sections on the following:

- **Roles**: The specific responsibilities of each member of the team, including the leader, should be delineated.
- **Discussion**: The manner in which discussion is to be held (agenda driven, Robert's rules of order, or open discussion) should be outlined.
- **Time**: The amount of time that members are expected to commit to team activities should be stated, including time for meetings.
- **Conduct**: Acceptable parameters for behavior should be clarified, including those for the individual and the group.
- **Conflict resolution**: Triggers for conflict resolution and methods should be agreed upon.
- **Reports**: The types of reports, timeline, and responsibility for preparing the reports must be clear.
- **Consequences**: Failure to follow the contract should result in consequences that are clearly identified.

### *Team Structure*

The appropriate team structure is very important in performance improvement because creating a team does not in itself ensure teamwork. The team must comprise individuals whose skills complement each other and who have a shared purpose because outcomes will depend on the collaborative efforts of the group rather than individuals within the group. Accordingly, the collective team is accountable for outcomes rather than the individuals. When creating teams, important **elements of the team structure** must be considered:

- **Size**: Teams of <10 members are most effective.
- **Skills**: Team members should have complementary skills that encompass technical, problem solving, decision making, and interpersonal domains.
- **Performance goals**: Teams should be allowed a degree of autonomy in producing action plans for performance improvement, based on strategic goals and objectives.
- **Unified approach**: Teams should be created according to the model of performance improvement, but they should have some flexibility in working together.
- **Accountability**: Team members are collectively, rather than individually, accountable.

## Diversity, Equity, and Inclusion Advocacy

### Generational Differences

Generational differences may occur outside of the family, but they can cause significant conflict when they occur within the family, especially if an older adult lives with younger generations. While individuals differ widely, as a group, older adults tend to be more religious and conservative than younger adults. Attitudes toward sexuality, equality, race, lifestyle, music, and religion may be divergent to the point that conflicts occur. General characteristics related to different generations include:

- **Silent generation** (born before WWII): Tend to be rule-oriented, cautious, and value trustworthiness and keeping their word. They are practical and make decisions based on interest and opportunity.
- **Baby boomers** (born 1943 to 1960): Tend to be more self-centered but proactive and committed to ideas/causes but resistant to compromise with others. They are focused on self-expression and introspection. This generation enjoyed prosperity to a greater degree than previous generations and came to expect that this prosperity would continue. They also had more access to health care and more medical tools (antibiotics, chemotherapy, and radiation).
- **Generation X** (born in the 1960s and 1970s): Tend to be independent in thoughts and lifestyle, are creative, and adapt well to change, but they may overlook ethical concerns in their quest for achievement. This generation was influenced by divorce more than were preceding generations. They seek balance and like to remain open to new opportunities.
- **Millennial (Y) generation** (born 1980 to 2000): Tend to believe they can be successful and are hardworking and confident in their abilities but may overlook the feelings and skills of others. They believe in the power of achievement and tend to make decisions as a family and are often more open to diversity (sexual preference, gender, race, culture) than previous generations.

## Health Literacy

Health literacy is the ability to obtain, understand, and consent to medical care to be able to make informed healthcare decisions, and health literacy must be considered when developing activities. Health literacy includes:

- Reading with comprehension, applying reason to context
- Understanding graphs and other visual representations of information
- Using the computer to obtain information
- Understanding the results of laboratory/radiographic studies
- Understanding and using basic mathematical computations
- Articulating concerns and questions
- Understanding basic anatomy and physiology
- Having basic knowledge of disease
- Understanding preventive health measures
- Knowing how to access health care and health information

Health literacy may be impacted by a number of factors, including lack of adequate education (low reading level), illiteracy, dementia, and learning disabilities. Those most vulnerable include elderly individuals, ethnic minorities, immigrants, and those with low income and/or chronic medical or physical health problems.

## Cultural Considerations

### *Hmong Patients*

The Hmong culture originates from Asian descent. The following considerations should be made when working with Hmong patients:

- The eldest male in the family makes the decisions for the family and is deferred to by other family members, so the nurse should ask who should receive information about the patient.
- Communication should be polite and respectful, avoiding direct eye contact, which is considered rude.
- Disagreeing is considered rude so "Yes" may mean "I hear you" and NOT "I agree with you."

### *Hispanic Patients*

Many areas of the country have large populations of Hispanics and Hispanic Americans. As always, it's important to recognize that cultural generalizations don't always apply to individuals. Recent immigrants, especially, have cultural needs that the nurse must understand:

- Many Hispanics are Catholic and may like the nurse to make arrangements for a priest to visit.
- Large extended families may come to visit to support the patient and family, so patients should receive clear explanations about how many visitors are allowed, but some flexibility may be required.
- Language barriers may exist as some may have limited or no English skills, so translation services should be available around the clock.
- Hispanic culture encourages outward expressions of emotions, so family may react strongly to news about a patient's condition, and people who are ill may expect some degree of pampering, so extra attention to the patient/family members may alleviate some of their anxiety.

**Caring for Hispanic and Hispanic American patients** requires understanding of cultural differences:

- Some immigrant Hispanics have very little formal education, so medical information may seem very complex and confusing, and they may not understand the implications or need for follow-up care.
- Hispanic culture perceives time with more flexibility than American culture, so if parents need to be present at a particular time, the nurse should specify the exact time (1:30 PM) and explain the reason rather than saying something more vague, such as "after lunch."
- People may appear to be unassertive or unable to make decisions when they are simply showing respect to the nurse by being deferent.
- In traditional families, the males make decisions, so a woman waits for the father or other males in the family to make decisions about treatment or care.
- Families may choose to use folk medicines instead of Western medical care or may combine the two.
- Children and young women are often sheltered and are taught to be respectful to adults, so they may not express their needs openly.

### *Middle Eastern Patients*

There are considerable cultural differences among Middle Easterners, but religious beliefs about the segregation of males and females are common. It's important to remember that segregating the female is meant to protect her virtue. Female nurses have low status in many countries because they violate this segregation by touching male bodies, so parents may not trust or show respect for the nurse who is caring for their family member. Additionally, male patients may not want to be cared for by female nurses or doctors, and families may be very upset at a female being cared for by a male nurse or physician. When possible, these cultural traditions should be accommodated:

- In Middle Eastern countries, males make decisions, so issues for discussion or decision should be directed to males, such as the father or spouse, and males may be direct in stating what they want, sometimes appearing demanding.
- If a male nurse must care for a female patient, then the family should be advised that *personal care* (such as bathing) will be done by a female while the medical treatments will be done by the male nurse.

**Caring for Middle Eastern patients** requires understanding of cultural differences:

- Families may practice strict dietary restrictions, such as avoiding pork and requiring that animals be killed in a ritual manner, so vegetarian or kosher meals may be required.
- People may have language difficulties requiring a translator, and same-sex translators should be used if at all possible.
- Families may be accompanied by large extended families that want to be kept informed and whom patients consult before decisions are made.
- Most medical care is provided by female relatives, so educating the family about patient care should be directed at females (with female translators if necessary).
- Outward expressions of grief are considered as showing respect for the dead.
- Middle Eastern families often offer gifts to caregivers. Small gifts (candy) that can be shared should be accepted graciously, but for other gifts, the families should be advised graciously that accepting gifts is against hospital policy.
- Middle Easterners often require less personal space and may stand very close.

### Asian Patients

There are considerable differences among different Asian populations, so cultural generalizations may not apply to all, but nurses caring for Asian patients should be aware of common cultural attitudes and behaviors:

- Nurses and doctors are viewed with respect, so traditional Asian families may expect the nurse to remain authoritative and to give directions and may not question, so the nurse should ensure that they understand by having them review material or give demonstrations and should provide explanations clearly, anticipating questions that the family might have but may not articulate.
- Disagreeing is considered impolite. "Yes" may only mean that the person is heard, not that they agree with the person. When asked if they understand, they may indicate that they do even when they clearly do not so as not to offend the nurse.
- Asians may avoid eye contact as an indication of respect. This is especially true of children in relation to adults and of younger adults in relation to elders.

**Caring for Asian patients** requires understanding of cultural differences:

- Patients/families may not show outward expressions of feelings/grief, sometimes appearing passive. They also avoid public displays of affection. This does not mean that they don't feel, just that they don't show their feelings.
- Families often hide illness and disabilities from others and may feel ashamed about illness.
- Terminal illness is often hidden from the patient, so families may not want patients to know they are dying or seriously ill.
- Families may use cupping, pinching, or applying pressure to injured areas, and this can leave bruises that may appear as abuse, so when bruises are found, the family should be questioned about alternative therapy before assumptions are made.
- Patients may be treated with traditional herbs.
- Families may need translators because of poor or no English skills.
- In traditional Asian families, males are authoritative and make the decisions.

## Conflict Resolution

### Positive and Negative Effects of Conflict

Some type of conflict is usually inevitable in any group of individuals, and it should be viewed as an opportunity for reflection rather than a failing. In fact, there are both negative and positive effects of conflict:

- **Negative**: Conflict can result in impaired communication and resentment and can damage the cohesiveness of a group of individuals, especially if people begin to take sides. Heated disagreements can escalate to fighting and aggressive behavior, and this can hinder performance.
- **Positive**: Conflict can result in new ideas and improved decision-making. Conflict can also result in increased creativity as individuals search for answers to the conflict and may bring about awareness for a need for better communication. Conflict can also result in increased interest and can provide a means of release of tension.

Conflict is best dealt with openly because unresolved conflicts can begin to mushroom into serious problems.

## Levels of Conflict

There are two primary levels of conflict:

- **Intrapersonal**: This type of conflict occurs within the individual, often when there are two competing needs or unmet needs. This can occur if a nurse is unhappy with an assignment or feels unable to provide the type of care desired because of job restrictions or inadequate staffing. This can manifest as withdrawal or anger.
- **Interpersonal**: This type of conflict occurs between or among individuals or groups. A typical example is a disagreement between a nurse and a doctor or between two nurses over issues of patient care or personal matters. Subtypes of interpersonal conflict include intragroup, intergroup, and interorganizational conflicts, such as disagreement between two departments and between nurses and doctors. A group may be splintered by different opinions Intergroup and interorganizational conflict may be difficult to resolve, especially if many people are involved, because of competing interests, and may require mediation.

## Types of Conflict

The three primary types of conflict include:

- **Relationship**: This is characterized by interpersonal conflicts that revolve around personal feelings and discord, such as a disagreement between two individuals. When relationship conflict is present, this can have a profoundly negative effect on team satisfaction and function, especially because people tend to become polarized, supporting one position or the other.
- **Task**: This is characterized by differences of opinions in how to accomplish a task, and it can result in heated discussions, but it rarely degenerates into negativity in the same way that relationship conflict does. Resolution should be evidence-based as much as possible.
- **Process**: This is characterized by differences of opinion about who is responsible for accomplishing a task. For example, group members may disagree about who is responsible for ordering supplies. This type of conflict is usually the easiest to resolve by compromise.

## Sources of Organizational Conflict

Conflict within an organization can occur for a number of reasons:

- **Power conflicts**: One party holds more power (such as physicians vs nurses, administrators vs. staff) and exercises this power, resulting in resentment and/or disagreement.
- **Impaired communication**: Parties may have a misunderstanding or may hold opposing views and are unable to discuss problems dispassionately.
- **Different goals**: Parties may have different goals, especially if the organizational goals are not clearly defined. Parties may have difference of opinions over general organizational policies.
- **Resource allocation**: Competition for the same or limited resources may lead to ongoing discord, especially if it appears that resources are allocated unfairly.
- **Role conflict**: Parties may suffer from role overload, the feeling that they are burdened with doing jobs that should be done by others. Parties may also have differing ideas about what roles entail.
- **Interpersonal conflicts**: Conflicts between individuals over personal matters can have broad impact. Sometimes, personal behavior by an individual is disturbing or upsetting to others.

## Ethical and Clinical Conflicts

Ethical and clinical conflicts among patients and their families and healthcare professionals are not uncommon. Issues frequently relate to medications and treatment, religion, concepts of truth telling, lack of respect for patient's autonomy, and limitations of managed care or incompetent care. Additionally, healthcare providers are in a position to easily manipulate patients/families by providing incomplete information to influence decisions, and this can give rise to ethical conflicts. Facilitation involves questioning and listening, acknowledging each person's perspective, while sharing different viewpoints:

- Open communication is critical to solving conflicts. Asking what steps could be taken to resolve the conflict or how it could be handled differently often leads to compromise because it allows for exchange of ideas and validates legitimate concerns. Sharing cultural perspectives can lead to better understanding.
- Advocacy for the patients/families must remain at the center of conflict resolution.

## Steps to Conflict Resolution in Teams

Conflict is an almost inevitable product of teamwork, and the leader must assume responsibility for **conflict resolution.** While conflicts can be disruptive, they can produce positive outcomes by opening dialogue and forcing team members to listen to different perspectives. The team should make a plan for dealing with conflict. The best time for conflict resolution is when differences emerge but before open conflict and hardening of positions occur. The leader must pay close attention to the people and problems involved, listen carefully, and reassure those involved that their points of view are understood. Steps to conflict resolution include:

- Allow both sides to present their side of conflict without bias, maintaining a focus on opinions rather than individuals.
- Encourage cooperation through negotiation and compromise.
- Maintain the focus, providing guidance to keep the discussions on track and avoid arguments.
- Evaluate the need for re-negotiation, formal resolution process, or third-party involvement.
- Utilize humor and empathy to diffuse escalating tensions.
- Summarize the issues, outlining key arguments.
- Avoid forcing resolution if possible.

## Conflict Management Approaches

Approaches to conflict resolution are as follows:

| | |
|---|---|
| **Accommodating** | One party ceding to the other, usually when the other has more power. |
| **Avoiding** | Taking steps to avoid dealing with the conflict. |
| **Collaborating** | Trying to find a solution that pleases both parties. |
| **Competing** | One party trying to win at all costs. |
| **Compromising** | Each party ceding something in return for harmony. |
| **Confronting** | Using "I" messages and assertive problem-solving. |
| **Forcing** | One party issuing orders to force a solution. |
| **Negotiating** | Similar to collaborating with back and forth bargaining. |
| **Reassuring** | Attempting to make everyone happy. |
| **Problem-solving** | Trying to find a solution that works for everyone using a step-by-step approach. |

| Withdrawing | One party withdrawing from the conflict, leaving the conflict unresolved. |
|---|---|

### Defensive Mode of Conflict Management

The defensive mode of conflict management focuses on avoiding open conflict even though the underlying problem may remain unresolved. Defensive strategies may be used if more proactive strategies (such as compromise) have failed or to initially defuse a situation until other strategies can be employed. Defensive measures include:

- **Separating the parties to the conflict**: This can mean assigning them to different teams or to different shifts or work schedules with different days off in order to avoid contact between those in conflict.
- **Avoiding/Suppressing conflict**: The parties in conflict may choose to avoid discussing the issue or problems or may be advised to do so by supervisory personnel.
- **Ignoring the conflict**: The parties in conflict may agree to disagree and to set the conflict aside and deal with other issues.
- **Providing an indirect solution**: An organizational change may eliminate the basis for the conflict.

### Lateral Violence and Bullying in the Workplace

Lateral violence (or horizontal violence) is a form of bullying that occurs among colleagues, most often directed at one or more individuals. When a senior nurse repeatedly interrupts a new graduate, stressing the new graduate's lack of experience, this is essentially belittling behavior meant to intimidate the new graduate and may result in a lack of confidence on the new graduate's part. Lateral violence can include physical contact (such as hitting and shoving) but most often it involves verbal or nonverbal expressions of hostility and conflict, including defensive postures (folded arms) and gestures meant to show contempt (rolling the eyes). Lateral violence as a form of workplace bullying may include name-calling, sarcastic statements, blaming, ignoring other's concerns, making inappropriate jokes, and interfering with others' rights as well as punishing others inappropriately. Lateral violence may cause the victim to lose self-esteem, emotional control, and motivation.

## Professional Development

### Professional Practice

#### *Role Clarification (ROLES)*

The ROLES acronym can be utilized as a guide to role clarification:

- **Responsibilities**: These include the specific job description for the role and tasks to be completed.
- **Opportunities**: These are aspects of the role that are not clearly definable but can be explored if the individual wants to engage.
- **Lines of communication**: This relates to the chain of command and refers to relationships with those with whom the individual will communicate, including subordinates, peers, and supervisors.
- **Expectations**: The administration may have both implicit and explicit expectations of a role that may conflict with the expectations of the individual. It is important that any role ambiguity be clarified to prevent role strain.

- **Support**: Support may be clearly defined, such as an accounting department to assist with budgetary issues, or less so, such as receiving support from peers or a mentor. It is important for the organization to outline support services and for the individual to consider the type of support needed to fulfill a role.

### NDP's Scope of Practice and Standards

The nursing professional development (NPD) specialist must be licensed as a professional nurse and have a graduate degree in nursing or a related discipline (if the BSN is in nursing). The NPD specialist practices within the scope of practice and standards established by the state board of nursing regulations. The NPD specialist is expected to demonstrate ongoing professional development through advanced academic education (such as a doctorate degree); continuing education; and professional activities that can include authoring, giving presentations, and participating in local, state, and national professional organizations. The NPD specialist should participate in a range of career advancement activities, such as establishing a program of mentoring, participating in research, and seeking administrative positions in order to influence policy and engage in decision making. The NPD specialist must focus on the use of technology, evidence-based practice, accountability, teaching and learning styles, generational differences, a global audience, and interdisciplinary collaboration, as well as fiscal management techniques, such as cost avoidance.

### Personal Accountability and Delegation

Personal accountability is the obligation to assume responsibility for one's own acts. This includes understanding the legal ramifications of actions, including supervision. Accountability is an issue in delegation, because the person who delegates is personally accountable for the appropriateness of delegation and the subsequent supervision of the delegated task. Prior to delegating tasks, the nurse should assess the needs of the patients and determine the task that needs to be completed, assure that he or she can remain accountable and can supervise the task appropriately, and evaluate effective completion. The **five rights of delegation** include:

- **Right task:** The nurse should determine an appropriate task to delegate for a specific patient. This would not include tasks that require assessment or planning.
- **Right circumstance:** The nurse has considered the setting, resources, time factors, safety factors, and all other relevant information to determine the appropriateness of delegation. A task that is usually in one's scope (such as feeding a patient) may require assessment that makes it inappropriate to delegate (feeding a new stroke patient).
- **Right person:** The nurse is in the right position to choose the right person (by virtue of education/skills) to perform a task for the right patient.
- **Right direction:** The nurse provides a clear description of the task, the purpose, any limits, and expected outcomes.
- **Right supervision:** The nurse is able to supervise, intervene as needed, and evaluate performance of the task.

### Mentoring

Mentoring occurs in many different ways. The professional may establish one-on-one mentoring relationships. Just as often, taking the time to assist others on a one-time basis or working with groups of staff provides an opportunity for mentoring. Mentoring is a reciprocal activity because both mentor and the mentee benefit. Mentoring is central to the role of the nurse and can be incorporated into current practice without involving extensive added responsibilities or time commitments. All interactions with other staff are essentially mentoring opportunities. The nurse should make a conscious decision to view himself or herself as a mentor and actively consider the role of mentor whenever working with other staff, especially when the nurse can identify a purpose, such as assisting others to learn new skills or providing demonstrations. The nurse can assist others to deal with issues of diversity.

#### ELEMENTS THAT ENHANCE MENTORING

The nursing professional development specialist is in an ideal position to serve as a mentor, both informally and formally. There are a number of elements that enhance mentoring:

- **Nurturing**: Being supportive and interested in furthering the skills and education of the staff.
- **Providing clinical expertise**: Guiding the staff by demonstrating a personal commitment to excellence in provision of care.
- **Motivating others**: Encouraging others and supporting them throughout their careers.
- **Providing an example**: Teaching others by being a good example.
- **Listening**: Being nonjudgmental in discussions with others and listening to determine different perspectives and needs.
- **Providing feedback**: Being honest in evaluation and assisting others to improve care, providing feedback about how their practices affect patient outcomes.
- **Role modeling**: Providing assistance to others in gaining certification and understanding the role of the CNS.

### *COACHING*

Coaching is an important part of mentoring/preceptoring. Coaching can include specific training, providing career information, and confronting issues of concern. While individual safety is the primary consideration, coaching should be done in a manner that increases learner confidence and ability to self-monitor rather than in a punitive or critical manner. The nurse must develop confidence in his or her own ability to be assertive and confront issues directly in order to resolve conflicts and promote collaboration. Effective methods of coaching include:

- Giving positive feedback, stressing what the person is doing right.
- Using questioning to help the person recognize problem areas.
- Providing demonstrations and opportunities for question/answer periods.
- Providing regular progress reports so the person understands areas of concern.
- Assisting the person to establish personal goals for improvement.
- Providing resources to help the person master material

#### CAREER DEVELOPMENT AND CLINICAL ADVANCEMENT

The career development relationship is one in which a coach or mentor assists another to become a socialized member of an organization and to develop skills and knowledge that allow for clinical advancement. This type of coaching requires face-to face contact and can include teaching when appropriate, training, and counseling about career choices. The coach should help the individual develop a positive attitude toward the work environment and should ensure the individual has opportunities for professional growth through continuing nursing education. The coach may help the individual to obtain a mentor and should encourage relationships with peers. The coach should also encourage the individual to explore different career options in order to find the one best suited for the individual and to pursue further education not only toward a specific goal but as an act of lifelong learning.

### NETWORKING

Networking, creating a system of contacts throughout the health industry and healthcare community, not only helps a professional development nurse to find employment but also provides valuable professional resources. Networking should begin with professors and instructors while the nurse is still a student, through demonstration of competence. The nurse can cooperate with others involved in clinical tasks or research, gaining experience and credibility. Those involved in sales of medications and equipment are resources that can provide the nurse with current trends and changes. One of the most effective ways to network is to become involved in national organizations and to participate in conferences through attendance and conference presentations. The professional development nurse should make an effort to maintain periodic contact with those in an informal network by telephone, mail, or email, or social networking sites, such as LinkedIn and Facebook, but the nurse must use care not to violate confidentiality and privacy and should avoid posting negative statements. Personal and professional sites should be kept separate, and private sites should be password protected.

### CAREER PLANNING WITH THE SMART TECHNIQUE

Career planning is an ongoing endeavor that includes self-evaluation and goal setting in order to determine what path the individual wants to take for career advancement. The individual should develop both a short-term and a long-term career plan, determining where he or she wants to be at a point in the future, such as in five years. The individual should conduct a career search, including the job market for potential careers and costs of education. One way to determine goals and establish a plan is to utilize the SMART technique:

- **Specific**: Identify concrete actions, and desired results: "Employment as nursing instructor."
- **Measurable**: Describes assessment parameters: "Work full-time in university program."
- **Achievable**: Appropriate for person's scope of practice and situation: "Studies show need for nursing instructors and opportunities for employment, and grants available for students."
- **Relevant/Realistic**: Opportunities exist: "Local universities advertising for nursing instructors."
- **Time-framed**: Beginning and ending dates for meeting goals: "Achieve goal within 3 years."

### SUCCESSION PLANNING

The first step in succession planning should be to describe the behaviors, skills, and leadership qualities necessary for the role. The next steps include outlining the needs of the organization and developing a formal written succession plan. An organization should have plans in place for both emergency succession and planned. An internal candidate is usually selected for emergency succession because of the need for someone to immediately step into the position and to be familiar with the organizational structure and current demands of the position. The chosen candidate usually fulfills the position on a temporary basis until planned succession can occur. Plans for succession should always be in place so that transitions are not disruptive to the organization. Planned succession may focus on both internal and external candidates, depending on the needs of the organization.

### ADVOCACY

Nurse competencies under the ACCN Synergy model include **advocacy/moral agency**:

- **Advocacy** is working for the best interests of the patient despite personal values in conflict and assisting patients to have access to appropriate resources.
- **Agency** is openness and recognition of issues and a willingness to act.
- **Moral agency** is the ability to recognize needs and take action to influence the outcome of a conflict or decision.

The levels of advocacy/moral agency include:

- **Level 1:** This nurse works on behalf of the patient, assesses personal values, has awareness of patient's rights and ethical conflicts, and advocates for the patient when consistent with the nurse's personal values.
- **Level 3:** This nurse advocates for the patient/family, incorporates their values into the care plan even when they differ from the nurse's, and can utilize internal resources to assist patient/family with complex decisions.
- **Level 5:** This nurse advocates for patient/family despite differences in values and is able to utilize both internal and external resources to help to empower patient/family to make decisions.

**Review Video: Patient Advocacy**
Visit mometrix.com/academy and enter code: 202160

## FEEDBACK STRATEGIES

### PERFORMANCE FEEDBACK

The nursing professional development specialist is often required to supervise other staff, especially when delegating tasks or supervising skills, and should provide evaluation and feedback. Performance feedback may take a variety of forms. The point of feedback is to help the person to improve skills, so immediate verbal feedback is usually more useful than delayed written feedback, although the supervisory role usually requires both. Feedback should include both reference to current practice and practical advice. Although sometimes overlooked, positive feedback promotes self-esteem and is motivating and easier than negative feedback, but advising supervised staff of problem areas is critical to patient safety and to helping them improve performance. One can begin by describing the situation and making specific observations about the person's performance, such as "This is what I observed," without judgment. Questioning includes:

- "How did you feel about the outcomes/procedure/task?"
- "What could you have done differently?"
- "How can I help you?"

If negligence requires disciplinary action, then the person should be provided the written policy.

### EFFECTIVE FEEDBACK FOR CRUCIAL CONVERSATIONS

Effective feedback strategies for crucial conversations include:

- Be objective and specific about the issue so that the individual is very clear about the issue of discussion.
- Communicate clearly and dispassionately, avoiding judgmental statements.

- Provide both positive and negative feedback rather than focusing only on the negative even if the primary issue is negative.
- Give feedback immediately, whether positive or negative.
- Provide frequent constructive feedback both publicly and privately.
- Give negative feedback only in private and maintain confidentiality so the individual can avoid embarrassment and others cannot overhear and draw inaccurate conclusions.
- Provide feedback based on observed behavior, with specific descriptions rather than generalities.
- Encourage the individual to also give feedback and express feelings.
- Provide suggestions for change (if the issue is simple) or methods to use to find a solution to a problem (if the issue is more complex).

### *TIMELINESS OF FEEDBACK*

Timeliness is a critical element of feedback. Studies have shown that immediate feedback is much more effective than delayed feedback. Feedback may be informal, such as when telling an individual that a job was well done or when suggesting alternative methods of solving a problem, or formal, such as when an individual meets with a supervisor to review job performance. Feedback is often more meaningful to the individual if given immediately; and, if feedback is delayed until a later time, the individual may have forgotten the incident or important details. Delayed feedback can also exacerbate conflict, especially if others are involved in the issue that needs to be resolved. While feedback often focuses on that which is negative, positive feedback is equally important and is a strong motivating factor when given frequently and consistently.

## FACILITATING GROUPS

### *INTERPROFESSIONAL/INTERDISCIPLINARY TEAMS*

There are a number of skills that are needed to lead and facilitate coordination of **intra- and inter-disciplinary teams:**

- Communicating openly is essential. All members must be encouraged to participate as valued members of a cooperative team.
- Avoiding interrupting or interpreting the point another is trying to make allows free flow of ideas.
- Avoiding jumping to conclusions, which can effectively shut off communication.
- Active listening requires paying attention and asking questions for clarification rather than to challenge other's ideas.
- Respecting others' opinions and ideas, even when opposed to one's own, is absolutely essential.
- Reacting and responding to facts rather than feelings allows one to avoid angry confrontations and diffuse anger.
- Clarifying information or opinions stated can help avoid misunderstandings.
- Keeping unsolicited advice out of the conversation shows respect for others and allows them to solicit advice without feeling pressured.

### *FOCUS GROUPS*

Focus groups provide a valuable tool for assessing customer needs. Focus groups of participants (8-12) are chosen because they share characteristics (age, ethnic background, community affiliation, health history, healthcare providers). The group usually meets for 1.5-2 hours for a focused discussion on a particular topic led by a facilitator or moderator with a recorder present and sometimes behind a one-way mirror. Nontraditional focus groups are sometimes conducted by conference telephone calls, internet groups, or videoconferences. Focus groups are told the topic before the discussion, and often begin by sharing stories. For example, if emergency care is the focus, then all might talk about their experiences in an emergency department. Then, the facilitator asks the group to focus on a few aspects of some stories in detail, and the stories are retold, with the facilitator using questions to prompt for more details. The group is asked to respond to the stories, including reactions, comments, and questions. A transcript of the meeting should be prepared for study.

### GROUP MEETINGS

Leading and facilitating groups requires utilizing good **techniques for meetings**. Considerations include:

- **Scheduling**: Both the time and the place must be convenient and conducive to working together, so the leader must review the work schedules of those involved, finding the most convenient time. Venues or meeting rooms should allow for sitting in a circle or around a table to facilitate equal exchange of ideas. Any necessary technology, such as computers or overhead projectors, or other equipment, such as whiteboards, should be available.
- **Preparation**: The leader should prepare a detailed agenda that includes a list of items for discussion.
- **Conduction**: Each item of the agenda should be discussed, soliciting input from all group members. Tasks should be assigned to individual members based on their interest and part in the process in preparation for the next meeting. The leader should summarize input and begin a tentative future agenda.
- **Observation**: The leader should observe the interactions, including verbal and nonverbal communication, and respond to them.

### PHASES OF THE GROUP PROCESS

Phases of the group process are as follows:

| | | |
|---|---|---|
| 1 | **Orientation** | Task is identified and members learn mission, depending primarily on the leader in the beginning, but members start to explore their own roles in the group and accept that change can occur. |
| 2 | **Organization** | Members make group decisions about rules, limits, criteria, and division of labor. Some resistance or fear of change may occur as members doubt the possibility of change, but members gain confidence as work of group becomes better organized. |
| 3 | **Flow of information** | Members become more able to express feelings and opinions and accept their roles in the group as interpersonal conflict lessons and group cohesion increases. |
| 4 | **Problem solving** | Members have a clear idea of task and are able to work collaboratively and interdependently. They feel satisfaction with the group and have confidence regarding reaching goals. However, some members or groups may reach an impasse and decide that goals cannot be met and actively resist change. |

### *Tuckman's Group Development Stages*

Tuckman's (1965) group developmental stages include:

- **Forming**: Group director takes more of an active role while members take their cues from the leader for structure and approval. The leader lists the goals and rules and encourages communication among the members.
- **Storming**: This stage involves a divergence of opinions regarding management, power, and authority. This stage may involve increased stress, and resistance may occur as shown by the absence of members, shared silence, and subgroup formation. At this point, the leader should promote and allow healthy expression of anger.
- **Norming**: It is at this stage where members express positive feelings toward each other and feel deeply attached to the group.
- **Performing**: The leader's input and direction decreases and mainly consists of keeping the group on course.
- **Mourning**: This is most deeply felt in closed groups when discontinuation of the group nears and in open groups when the leader or other members leave.

# Ethical, Legal, and Regulatory Standards

## Professional Standards, Certification, and Credentialing

### Obtaining Information Regarding Certification

Information about certifications can be obtained from a number of different sources:

- **State boards of nursing**: Each state outlines the type of certifications recognized for advance practice nurses and provides the scope of practice.
- **Books**: Career-related nursing books are widely available regarding all different types of certifications.
- **Journals**: Nursing journals often have career-related articles and/or articles of interest to those with specific certifications. Other journals are aimed at those with certification in a specific field, such as the *Clinical Journal of Oncology Nursing*, and can provide valuable insight into the specialized practice.
- **State and national professional organizations**: Organizations such as the National Nursing Staff Development Organization provide information about certification programs, including location of programs, professional resources, and requirements.
- **Certification organizations**: Organizations that provide credentialing, such as the American Nurses Credentialing Center (ANCC), provide information about obtaining certification, maintaining, and renewing.

### Coordinating Certification and Credentialing

When coordinating activities that support certification and credentialing, the nursing professional development specialist must first determine the type of certification and credentialing and the specific requirements of the credentialing organization in order to produce activities that can be counted toward achieving or maintaining certification and credentialing. The nurse must provide oversight to ensure that certification activities are performed effectively and documented as required. Coordinating responsibilities include:

- Providing adequate support system
- Developing educational programs and activities or assisting and supervising others to do so
- Developing educational materials in support of certification/credentialing
- Collecting data regarding certification/credentialing and maintaining records
- Consulting with professionals as needed to facilitate activities
- Managing budget for activities
- Initiating programs for quality performance improvement
- Auditing individual records of educational activities and preparing reports
- Communicating with staff personally or via telephone and/or email to respond to questions regarding activities

### Licensure

While accreditation processes are voluntary, licensure is mandatory, usually through the State Department of Health Services. Organizations must be in compliance with state and federal laws and regulations in order to be licensed. Managed care organizations are usually licensed by other state departments, such as the Department of Insurance. There are a number of different **types of licenses**, and these may vary slightly from one state to another:

- Acute medical and psychiatric hospitals
- Ambulatory surgical centers
- Skilled nursing facilities and subacute care centers
- Long-term care facilities
- Home health care agencies
- Hospice agencies
- Assisted living programs
- Residential programs for behavioral/mental/developmentally disabled

Organizations that use beds or staffing in ways that are noncompliant risk losing their licenses. Licenses specify the number of patient beds and types of patients as well as staffing provisions, which may vary from state to state.

## Professional Documentation Requirements

### *Purposes of Documentation*

Documentation is a form of communication that provides information about the patient and confirms that care was provided. Accurate, objective, and complete documentation of individual care is required by both accreditation and reimbursement agencies, including federal and state governments. **Purposes of documentation** include:

- Carrying out professional responsibility
- Establishing accountability
- Communicating among healthcare professionals
- Educating staff
- Providing information for research
- Satisfying legal and practice standards
- Ensuring reimbursement

While patient care documentation focuses on progress notes, there are many other aspects to charting. Doctor's orders must be noted, medication administration must be documented on medication sheets or in the electronic health system's MAR, and vital signs must be graphed. Flow sheets must be checked off, filled out, or initialed. Admission assessments may involve primarily checklists or may require extensive documentation. The primary issue in malpractice cases is inaccurate or incomplete documentation. It is better to over-document than under, but effective documentation does neither.

### *Accuracy in Documentation*

There are a number of requirements regarding written communication and documentation, including accuracy. Regardless of format, patient care charting should always include any change in client's condition, any treatments, medications, or other interventions, client responses, and any complaints of family or client. Nurses should avoid subjective descriptions (especially negative terms, which could be used to establish bias in court), such as tired, angry, confused, bored, rude, happy, and euphoric. Instead, more objective descriptions, such as "yawning 2-3 times a minute," should be used. Clients can be quoted directly, "I shouldn't have to wait for pain medication when I need it!" If errors are made in paper charting, for example, charting another patient's information in the record, the error cannot be erased, whited-out, or otherwise made illegible. The error must be indicated by drawing a line through the text and writing "Error."

### TIMELINESS OF DOCUMENTATION

Written communication/documentation requirements also include timeliness. Nurses should chart every 1-2 hours for routine care (bathing, walking), but medications and other interventions or changes in condition should be charted immediately. Failure to chart medications, especially as-needed (PRN) medications, in a timely manner may result in the client receiving the medication twice. Additionally, if one nurse is caring for a number of patients, it may be easy to forget and omit or confuse information. Nurses must never chart in advance because it is illegal and can lead to unforeseen errors. Guessing that a client will have no problems and care will be routine can result in having to make corrections. Nurses must chart the time of all interventions and notations. Time may be a critical element, for example, in deciding if a patient should receive more pain medication or be catheterized for failure to urinate. Military time is used in many healthcare institutions but if standard time is used, the nurse should always include "AM" or "PM" with time notations.

### LEGIBILITY AND CLARITY OF DOCUMENTATION

Additional written communication/documentation requirements include:

- **Legibility**: If hand entries are used, then writing should be done with a blue or black permanent ink pen, and writing should be neat and legible, in block printing if handwriting is illegible. Some facilities require black ink only, so if unsure, nurses should use black ink. No pen or pencil that can be erased can be used to document in a patient's record because this could facilitate falsification of records. For the same reason, a line must be drawn through empty spaces in the documentation.
- **Clarity**: A standardized vocabulary should be used for documenting, including lists of approved abbreviations and symbols. Abbreviations and symbols, especially, can pose serious problems in interpretation, so they should be used sparingly.

### METHODS OF DOCUMENTATION

Different methods of documentation include the following:

- **Flow sheets**: These are often a part of other methods of charting and are used to save time. Electronic health record platforms often have flow sheets embedded into their documentation system and the ability to automatically convert charted data (such as vital signs) into charts/graphs which visually depict trends in the patient's health and progress. Flow sheets may also be used to indicate completion of exercises or treatments. They usually contain areas for graphing data and may have columns or rows with information requiring checkmarks to indicate an action was done or observation made.
- **Critical pathways**: These are specific multidisciplinary care plans that outline interventions and outcomes of diseases, conditions, and procedures. Critical pathways are based on data and literature and best practices. The expected outcomes are delineated as well as the sequence of interventions and the timeline needed to achieve the outcomes. There are many different types of forms that appear similar to flow sheets but are more complex and require more documentation. Any variance from the pathway or expected outcomes must be documented. Critical pathways are increasingly used to comply with insurance limitations to ensure cost-effective timely treatment.

### RECORD RETENTION

The duration of record retention depends on the specific record as well as state, accreditation, or federal regulations. In general, health records of individuals should usually be retained for 10 years or until the age of maturity for minors as specified by the state. Some records, such as registers of births, deaths, and surgical procedures, must be maintained permanently. Other records, such as images, must be maintained for five years. Records of continuing education must be retained in accordance with state laws or certifying agency requirements. When paper records no longer need to be retained, they must be destroyed by shredding and/or incinerating. Because electronic health records can be stored easily and are relatively inexpensively, some organizations have chosen to simply save them permanently; however, hardware and software obsolescence may present problems in retrieving electronic records after they have been saved. This may require periodically making new copies of old records.

# Scope of Practice and Code of Ethics

## Legal Issues Related to Working Outside of One's Scope of Practice

Depending on the seriousness of the issue related to scope of practice, the nurse may report violations of legal and regulatory requirements to an immediate supervisor or other supervisory person, according to established protocol, or directly to a regulatory agency. In almost all cases, regulatory agencies, such as OSHA, provide a method (online, fax, mail, telephone) to file a confidential complaint and protect the person from reprisals, such as firing or demotion. Some types of issues have a timeline, so reports should be completed immediately when the nurse becomes aware of violations. Additionally, each state has regulatory boards that are responsible for investigating violations of legal and regulatory standards, and these regulatory boards should investigate and take action after a complaint is filed. There are specific federal and state regulations regarding breaches of confidentiality regarding health information, requiring individuals, HHS, and the media (if more than 500 individuals involved) to be notified.

## ANA Nursing Code of Ethics

The American Nurse Association (ANA) developed the **Nursing Code of Ethics.** There are nine provisions:

1. The nurse treats all patients with respect and consideration, regardless of social circumstances or health condition.
2. The nurse's primary commitment is to the patient regardless of conflicts that may arise.
3. The nurse promotes and advocates for the patient's health, safety, and rights, while maintaining privacy and confidentiality and protecting patients from questionable practices or care.
4. The nurse is responsible for his or her own care practices and determine appropriate delegation of care.
5. The nurse must retain respect for self and his or her own integrity and competence.
6. The nurse participates in ensuring that the healthcare environment is conducive to providing good health care and consistent with professional and ethical values.
7. The nurse participates in education and knowledge development to advance the profession.
8. The nurse collaborates with others to promote efforts to meet health needs.
9. The nursing profession articulates values and promotes and maintains the integrity of the profession.

## Ethical Considerations

### *Ethical Principles*

**Beneficence** is an ethical principle that involves performing actions that are for the purpose of benefitting another person. In the care of a patient, any procedure or treatment should be done with the ultimate goal of benefitting the patient, and any actions that are not beneficial should be reconsidered. As conditions change, procedures need to be continually reevaluated to determine if they are still of benefit.

**Nonmaleficence** is an ethical principle that means healthcare workers should provide care in a manner that does not cause direct intentional harm to the patient:

- The actual act must be good or morally neutral.
- The intent must be only for a good effect.
- A bad effect cannot serve as the means to get to a good effect.
- A good effect must have more benefit than a bad effect has harm.

**Autonomy** is the ethical principle that the individual has the right to make decisions about his or her own care. In the case of children or patients with dementia who cannot make autonomous decisions, parents or family members may serve as the legal decision maker. The nurse must keep the patient and/or family fully informed so that they can exercise their autonomy in informed decision-making.

**Justice** is the ethical principle that relates to the distribution of the limited resources of healthcare benefits to the members of society. These resources must be distributed fairly. This issue may arise if there is only one bed left and two sick patients. Justice comes into play in deciding which patient should stay and which should be transported or otherwise cared for. The decision should be made according to what is best or most just for the patients and not colored by personal bias.

### *Informed Consent*

Patients or guardians must provide informed consent for all treatment the patient receives. This includes a thorough explanation of all procedures and treatment and associated risks. Patients/guardians should be apprised of all options and allowed input on the type of treatments. Patients/guardians should be apprised of all reasonable risks and any complications that might be life threatening or increase morbidity. The American Medical Association has established **guidelines for informed consent:**

- Explanation of diagnosis
- Nature of, and reason for, treatment or procedure
- Risks and benefits
- Alternative options (regardless of cost or insurance coverage)
- Risks and benefits of alternative options
- Risks and benefits of not having a treatment or procedure
- Providing informed consent is a requirement of all states

Note: A patient may waive their right to informed consent; if this is the case, the nurse should document the patient's refusal and proceed with the procedure. Also, informed consent is not necessary for procedures performed to save a life/limb in which the patient/family is unable to consent.

### *Bioethics*

Bioethics is a branch of ethics that involves making sure that the medical treatment given is the most morally correct choice given the different options that might be available and the differences inherent in the varied levels of treatment. In the health care unit, if the patients, family members, and the staff are in agreement when it comes to values and decision-making, then no ethical dilemma exists; however, when there is a difference in value beliefs between the patients/family members and the staff, there is a bioethical dilemma that must be resolved. Sometimes, discussion and explanation can resolve differences, but at times the institution's ethics committee must be brought in to resolve the conflict. The primary goal of bioethics is to determine the most morally correct action using the set of circumstances given.

### *Ethical Implications of Resource Allocation*

Resource allocation in healthcare is an ethical issue that is not easily resolved. Perspectives include:

- **Right to care**: If all patients deserve an equal right to care but resources are limited, then the task becomes one of determining ways to acquire more resources so that all can be served, but this is not always possible. There is unequal geographic and economic distribution of resources.
- **Quality of life**: If limited resources are allocated according to quality-of-life issues, someone has to decide what qualities take precedence, but there is little consensus in health care. Gender, race, and ethnicity should not be factors, but it can be difficult to separate these from economic factors or social support issues.
- **Economic considerations**: With limited resources, care is often rationed according to those who have insurance or other economic means to pay for care. Medicaid and other programs to pay for care provide some balance, but these programs may not pay for expensive procedures that are available to those with more financial resources.

### *Environmental Ethics*

Environmental ethics focus on the belief that human beings have an ethical obligation to the environment and that ethical considerations should be applied to the environment as well as to living things. This includes such things as consideration of the carbon footprint of not only individuals and groups but organizations and governments. Environmental ethics focuses on protection of the environment and prevention of damage and recognizes that all things, living and nonliving, are related and affect each other, negatively or positively. Environmental ethics extends moral standings to animals as well. When applying environmental ethics to healthcare organizations, considerations include:

- Reducing waste and recycling materials
- Reducing heating/cooling use through better construction practices
- Providing appropriate waste management
- Using environmentally friendly materials in construction
- Identifying alternative products to those that contain toxins or harmful substances
- Preventing downstream pollution from medical waste

## Professional Boundaries

Professional boundaries that show respect for the individual can be difficult to establish as part of delivery of care, especially with diverse populations because the nurse may unknowingly violate personal or spiritual values. Diverse groups include those on the fringes of society, such as the homeless or the abused. It is very important that nurses remain cognizant of the potential to abuse a position of power in which the individual and family are in many ways dependent upon the nurse. Also, because of language barriers, fears, or cultural constraints, the individual and family may not feel able to state their concerns. A relationship with an individual must be caring but at the same time professional and nonjudgmental. The needs of the individual/family must always be considered, and this may mean using a translator to ensure that the individual/family are assuming an active role in the plan of care or making referrals to others in the healthcare or allied professions.

### Commercial Bias and Vested Interest

**Commercial bias** is showing preference for one commercial product or company over another because of personal feelings or personal benefit rather than evidence of quality. The nurse should take care to avoid promoting a particular product or service and should make full disclosure if a conflict of interest, such as a financial interest in company, occurs.

A **vested interest** occurs if the individual makes a decision based on the potential for financial or other gain. Disclosure should include any financial incentive/payment, the name of the company, and the person's relationship to the company. Commercial bias may be an issue if a close family member, such as a spouse or sibling, has an interest in a company as well. Recommendations should be based on evidence-based research, quality, and cost-effectiveness. When companies serve as a source of funding for programs or research, an institution must take extra steps to ensure that commercial bias does not affect outcomes/decisions and all those involved are aware of the potential for bias.

### Conflict of Interest

Conflict of interest occurs when an individual has a personal financial or nonfinancial interest that could result in bias or acting in self-interest. Types of conflicts of interest include:

- **Financial gain**: The individual profits because of an interest, such as when the person has ownership in a company doing business with the organization that employs the individual.
- **Nepotism**: The individual shows favoritism in hiring or promoting a family member or friend over better qualified applicants.
- **Employment**: The individual may be employed in a second job that is in conflict with the first.
- **Gift-receiving**: The individual accepts gifts from others who may, in turn, expect special consideration. This may include accepting gifts or gratuities for conducting a product evaluation.
- **Self-serving actions**: The individual alone profits from a transaction.
- **Royalties**: The individual may promote books or inventions for which the individual receives royalties.

### Intellectual Property

The two types of intellectual property include industrial property and copyrighted material.

- **Industrial property** includes inventions, designs (industrial), symbols, and names utilized in commercial endeavors. These belong to the owner and cannot be used without permission or, in the case of most inventions, purchase or contractual agreement. Patents and trademarks are considered intellectual property. Patents are granted for inventions after the inventor applies and submits a description that is available to the public. Trademarks, such as the Apple on Mac computers, require application and are used to identify goods and services.
- **Copyrighted material** includes literary and artistic works, such as books, articles, and other writings, and paintings, drawings, and photographs. Copyrighted materials are often used by others in research or articles and can be used with permission of the author or artist. Some exceptions allow "fair use" of materials without prior permission for research/scholarship, educational purposes, critical review, or journalism.

### Plagiarism

Plagiarism is an act of fraud that involves using others' words, ideas, expressions, or productions and presenting them as one's own rather than giving credit to the originator. While plagiarism itself is not considered a criminal act, it can in some cases involve copyright infringement, which is a criminal act. Plagiarism is considered academic dishonesty and may incur institutional punishment, such as being expelled from a program. Plagiarism can include:

- Stealing an entire work and presenting it as one's own
- Copying part of someone else's work without citation
- Failing to use quotation marks around a quotation
- Paraphrasing someone else's work directly
- Exceeding fair use of someone else's work, even with a citation
- Copying different types of media (illustrations, video, audio, and photos) without permission
- Using copyrighted music without permission for a soundtrack
- Including the music written by another person in a musical composition

### Cheating

Cheating is a dishonest means of achieving a goal or gaining recognition. In a professional setting, cheating can take many forms, such as falsifying records (time, academic, patient care), plagiarizing, copying exams, and taking credit for others' achievements. The best way to deal with cheating is to put safeguards in place to make cheating more difficult, including outlining potential consequences. When cheating is identified, it should be dealt with immediately in private, but the person confronting the person cheating should be prepared with proof because the first inclination people have when caught cheating is to deny: "You took credit for the work that Ms. Smith did on the quality improvement project. I have copies of the draft she prepared a week before you handed in the same report under your name." In some cases, cheating is a dismissible offense, but in other cases, milder consequences may apply. In either case, a discussion about the reason for cheating should take place.

### Sexual Boundaries

When the boundary between the role of the professional nurse and the vulnerability of the patient is breached, a boundary violation occurs. Because the nurse is in the position of authority, the responsibility to maintain the boundary rests with the nurse; however, the line separating them is a continuum and sometimes not easily defined. It is inappropriate for nurses to engage in **sexual relations** with patients, and if the sexual behavior is coerced or the patient is cognitively impaired, it is **illegal**. However, more common violations with adults, particularly elderly patients, include exposing a patient unnecessarily, using sexually demeaning gestures or language (including off-color jokes), harassment, or inappropriate touching. Touching should be used with care, such as touching a hand or shoulder. Hugging may be misconstrued.

### Gifts

Over time, patients may develop a bond with nurses they trust and may feel grateful to the nurse for the care provided and want to express thanks, but the nurse must make sure to maintain professional boundaries. Patients often offer **gifts** to nurses to show their appreciation, but some adults, especially those who are weak and ill or have cognitive impairment, may be taken advantage of easily. Patients may offer valuables and may sometimes be easily manipulated into giving large sums of money. Small tokens of appreciation that can be shared with other staff, such as a box of chocolates, are usually acceptable (depending upon the policy of the institution), but almost any other gifts (jewelry, money, clothes) should be declined: "I'm sorry, that's so kind of you, but nurses are not allowed to accept gifts from patients." Declining may relieve the patient of the feeling of obligation.

### Coercion

Power issues are inherent in matters associated with professional boundaries. Physical abuse is both unprofessional and illegal, but behavior can easily border on abusive without the patient being physically injured. Nurses can easily **intimidate** older adults and sick patients into having procedures or treatments they do not want. Regardless of age, patients have the right to choose and the right to refuse treatment. Difficulties arise with cognitive impairment, and in that case, another responsible adult (often the patient's child or spouse) is designated to make decisions, but every effort should be made to gain patient cooperation. Forcing the patient to do something against his or her will borders on abuse and can sometimes degenerate into actual abuse if physical coercion is involved.

### Attention

Nursing is a giving profession, but the nurse must temper giving with recognition of professional boundaries. Patients have many needs. As acts of kindness, nurses (especially those involved in home care) often give certain patients extra attention and may offer to do **favors**, such as cooking or shopping. They may become overly invested in the patients' lives. While this may benefit a patient in the short term, it can establish a relationship of increasing **dependency** and **obligation** that does not resolve the long-term needs of the patient. Making referrals to the appropriate agencies or collaborating with family to find ways to provide services is more effective. Becoming overly invested may be evident by the nurse showing favoritism or spending too much time with the patient while neglecting other duties. On the other end of the spectrum are nurses who are disinterested and fail to provide adequate attention to the patient's detriment. Lack of adequate attention may lead to outright neglect.

### Personal Information

When pre-existing personal or business relationships exist, other nurses should be assigned care of the patient whenever possible, but this may be difficult in small communities. However, the nurse should strive to maintain a professional role separate from the personal role and respect professional boundaries. The nurse must respect and maintain the confidentiality of the patient and family members, but the nurse must also be very careful about **disclosing personal information** about him or herself because this establishes a social relationship that interferes with the professional role of the nurse and the boundary between the patient and the nurse. The nurse and patient should never share secrets. When the nurse divulges personal information, he or she may become vulnerable to the patient, a reversal of roles.

## Organizational Accreditation

### Joint Commission

The Joint Commission is the primary accrediting agency for healthcare programs in the United States. The Joint Commission establishes accreditation standards for various types of healthcare programs, establishes general competencies for healthcare practitioners, and issues annual National Patient Safety Goals. Standards for accreditation are, for the most part, performance based and focus on measures of processes and outcomes and issues related to patient care and safety.

Comparative performance measure data, such as core measures, are integrated into the accreditation process. Most surveyors assess compliance based on the following:

- Document review to validate compliance
- Onsite inspections and observations
- Interviews of staff
- Review of standards implementation measures
- Review of medical records
- Assessment of service and support systems of the organization
- Integration of performance measure data

The surveyors may recommend denial of accreditation if conditions exist that pose a threat to staff, patients, or the public, but the organization may request the opportunity to demonstrate compliance through documentation or interviews, and in some cases a second survey may be conducted.

## National Committee for Quality Assurance (NCQA)

The National Committee for Quality Assurance (NCQA), a private nonprofit agency that accredits health plans, has addressed safety issues as part of its accreditation standards in response to the Institute of Medicine (IOM) call for accrediting agencies to ensure organizations focus on patient safety. Guidelines directed at managed care organizations provide useful information for other organizations as well. Organization should:

- Educate staff regarding clinical safety by providing information.
- Provide collaborative training within the network related to safe clinical practice.
- Combine data within the network (organization) on adverse outcomes/polypharmacy.
- Make improving patient safety a priority for quality improvement activities.
- Provide and distribute information about safe practices that includes information about computerized pharmacy order systems, intensive care trained physicians, best practices, research on safe clinical practices.

## Magnet Status

The American Nurse's Credentialing Center, affiliated with the ANA, developed the **Magnet Recognition Program** to reward hospitals that meet a set of criteria related to excellence in nursing and positive patient outcomes associated with high job satisfaction and low staff turnover. Hospitals must apply for Magnet status and undergo extensive review for compliance. Criteria include:

- Educational requirements: Chief nursing officer (CNO) must have MS or doctorate in nursing; 100% of nurse managers must have a degree in nursing (BS or higher) and 100% of nurse leaders must have a degree in nursing (BS or higher).
- Evidence of innovative health care.
- Patient outcome data: includes falls, pressure ulcers, BSI, UTI, VAP, restraint use, pediatric IV infiltrations, and other nationally benchmarked indicators of specific specialties. Data should outperform the mean of the selected national database.
- Patient satisfaction surveys and data: pain management, education, nursing courtesy and respect, listening, and response time.

# Risk Management

## Analysis and Avoidance

Risk management is an organized and formal method of decreasing liability, financial loss, and risk or harm to patients, staff, or others by doing an assessment of risk and introducing risk management strategies. Much of risk management has been driven by the insurance industry in order to minimize costs, but quality management utilizes risk management as a method to ensure quality health care and process improvement. An organization's risk management program usually comprises a manager and staff with a number of responsibilities:

- **Risk identification** begins with an assessment of processes to identify and prioritize those that require further study to determine risk exposure.
- **Risk analysis** requires a careful documenting of process, utilizing flow charts, with each step in the process assessed for potential risks. This may utilize root cause analysis methods.
- **Risk prevention/avoidance** involves instituting corrective or preventive processes. Responsible individual or teams are identified and trained.
- **Assessment/evaluation of corrective/preventive processes** is ongoing to determine if they are effective or require modification.

## Risk Stratification

Risk stratification involves statistical adjustment to account for confounding and differences in risk factors. Confounding issues are those that confuse the data outcomes, such as trying to compare different populations, different ages, or different genders. For example, if there are two physicians and one has primarily high-risk patients, and the other has primarily low-risk patients, the same rate of infection (by raw data) would suggest that the infection risks are equal for both physicians' patients. However, high-risk patients are much more prone to infection, so in this case risk stratification to account for this difference would show that the patients of the physician with low-risk patients had a much higher risk of infection, relatively speaking. Risk stratification is also used to predict outcomes of surgery by accounting for various risk factors (including ASO score, age, and medical conditions). Risk stratification is an important element of data/outcome analysis.

## Accountability

The nurse has an obligation to report ethical and standards of care violations and to intervene to ensure safety of the patient. This accountability is outlined by state boards of nursing, professional organizations, and accrediting agencies. The nurse must report suspected or observed diversion of drugs, any type of abuse (physical, emotional, sexual, financial), falsification of patient records, neglect of patients, narcotic offenses, and arrests, indictments, and/or convictions for criminal offenses. Each facility should have policies in place for reporting, but the usual procedure is to report to the immediate supervisor and file an incident report; however, the nurse can file a complaint directly with the board of nursing, especially if the matter is serious. The written report is essential in the event that the nurse should experience reprisals. After filing a report, the nurse should follow up to determine if action has been taken. With ethical dilemmas, a report may be made to the bioethics committee. Violations may result in disciplinary action, mentoring, or loss of license.

## Safety

Because risk management is concerned with decreasing liability and increasing safety, integrating the outcomes of risk management assessment into the performance improvement process requires an organization-wide commitment to reducing risk. The governing board and quality professional must ensure that the risk management assessments are considered when formulating mission and vision statements and strategic goals. During process evaluation and process improvement processes, risk management assessment should be one of the first concerns. An organization-wide early warning system should be in place to screen patients for potential risks and identify the following:

- **Adverse patient occurrences (APOs):** Those unexpected events that result in a negative impact on the patient's health or welfare.
- **Potentially compensable events (PCEs):** APOs that may result in claims against the organization because of the negative impact on the patient's health or welfare.

If the organization has set up a method to quickly identify problems, then risks may be minimized.

## Patient Safety Program

### *Development*

Each healthcare organization has unique needs and challenges to face in developing a patient safety program, although many components are universally needed. Facilitating development of a patient safety program requires planning and taking steps to include the following:

- Identifying a quality professional or interdisciplinary group to manage the safety program.
- Defining the scope of the program, including risk identification and management as well as response to adverse events.
- Providing mechanisms to integrate all aspects of the program into functions organization-wide.
- Establishing procedures for rapid response to medical errors or adverse events.
- Establishing procedures for both internal and external reporting of medical errors.
- Defining and disseminating intervention strategies such as risk reduction, tracking of risks, and root-cause analysis.
- Outlining mechanisms for staff support related to involvement in sentinel events.
- Establishing procedures and responsibilities for reporting to the governing board.

### *Components*

A quality patient safety program must include a number of different components:

- Functional infrastructure with leader, safety officer, teams, and software for tracking and measures.
- Linkage of program goals with strategic goals of the organization.
- Establishment of policies and procedures to reduce and control risk and supportive educational training.
- Reporting system to identify adverse events or incidents.
- Participation in national patient safety initiatives, such as NPSGs, IPSG, IHI 5 Million Lives, and Leapfrog.
- Rapid response procedures to deal with medical errors and sentinel events.
- Adequate data collection procedures to ensure performance measurement, tracking, and data analysis.
- Performance improvement activities directed at specific goals.
- Documentation of all processes and procedures and reporting procedures and timelines.

## Management of Environmental Safety Hazards and Risks

### Initial Steps

Development of a patient safety program must include evaluation and management of environmental safety hazards and risks. Environmental concerns include:

- Preparing a written plan that clearly outlines environmental safety concerns, policies, and procedures.
- Identifying security risks, such as infant/child abduction and establishing processes to increase security, such as the use of alarms, identification badges, locks, better lighting, and security officers.
- Evaluating power/utility requirements, including emergency power, and maintaining, testing, and inspecting utilities.
- Establishing an interdisciplinary team to identify opportunities for improvement and facilitate performance improvement processes.
- Completing risk assessment of physical plant, including buildings, grounds, equipment, and related systems, such as electrical, lighting, IT, ventilation, and plumbing.
- Establishing a plan for emergency preparedness, including evaluation of areas of vulnerability, preparedness, response, and recovery.

### Ongoing Efforts

A patient safety program must include ongoing evaluation and management of environmental safety hazards and risks:

- Establishing organization-wide safety policies and procedures, including no smoking policies.
- Maintaining the physical plant and monitoring and responding to product recalls.
- Handling, storing, and disposing of hazardous wastes, including identifying wastes that are corrosive, ignitable, reactive, or toxic, and following state and EPA regulations and educating staff.
- Conducting fire safety drills and checking equipment and buildings for fire dangers.
- Monitoring medical equipment, including ensuring routine maintenance, testing, and regular inspection.
- Establishing a safe environment for staff and patients, including fall prevention strategies, such as installing handrails, contrast strips on stairways, and analyzing work flow to facilitate functions.
- Designating individuals to monitor and coordinate environmental safety management and to develop procedures for dealing with threats/problems.

## National Patient Safety Goals

The Joint Commission issues National Patient Safety Goals annually for different types of healthcare programs, but the hospital goals are fairly representative:

- **Improve accuracy of patient identification**: Utilize two patient identifiers.
- **Improve the effectiveness of communication among caregivers**: Standards for abbreviations, "read back" for verbal or telephone orders, improved timeline for reporting test results
- **Improve the safety of using medications**: Proper labeling, review of drugs with similar names/appearances, reduction in anticoagulation therapy risks

- **Reduce the risk of healthcare-associated infections**: WHO or CDC handwashing guidelines and treating healthcare-associated infections as sentinel events
- **Accurately and completely reconcile medications across the continuum of care**: Accurate listing of patient's medications for patient and other providers
- **Reduce the risk of patient harm from falls**: Fall reduction program
- **Involve patients actively in their own care as a patient safety strategy**: Reporting of safety concerns
- **Identify inherent patient safety risks**: Includes risk of suicide
- **Improve recognition and response to changes in a patient's condition**: Immediate response, consultation

## National Quality Forum Safe Practices

The National Qualify Forum (NQF) has endorsed a set of safe practices that can be used to assess and develop the organization's patient safety culture. Practices encompass creating a safe culture as well as specific steps to ensure safe practices throughout the organization. According to NQF, the four elements needed to **create and sustain a patient safety culture** include:

- Leadership must ensure structures are in place for organization-wide awareness and compliance with safety measures, including adequate resources and direct accountability.
- Measurement, analysis, and feedback must track safety and allow for interventions.
- Team-based patient care with adequate training and performance improvement activities must be organization-wide.
- Safety risk must be continuously identified and interventions taken to reduce patient risk.

Additional concepts relevant to the National Quality Forum include the following:

- Considering the rights and responsibilities of the patient by providing informed consent, respecting advance directives and patients' directions related to care, and providing full disclosure of medical error.
- Providing adequate well-trained and supervised staff and resources to meet healthcare needs as well as critical care certified physicians for intensive care or critical care units.
- Managing information and care through documenting care properly, providing prompt accurate test results, utilizing standardized procedures for labeling diagnostic studies, and providing discharge planning.
- Managing medications by implementing a computerized prescriber order entry (CPOE) system, standardizing abbreviations, maintaining updated medication lists for patients, including pharmacists in medication management, including selecting a formulary, standardizing labeling, identifying high-alert drugs, and dispensing drugs in unit doses.
- Preventing healthcare-associated infections (HAIs) through ventilator bundle intervention, following best practices for central venous lines, complying with CDC handwashing guidelines, immunizing staff and patients for influenza, and preventing surgical site infections through the appropriate use of antibiotics, proper hair removal, glucose control for cardiac patients, and temperature control for colorectal surgery.
- Providing safe practices for surgery, such as informing patients of risks and taking measures to prevent errors such as operating on the wrong site, and use prophylactic treatments as indicated to prevent complications.
- Providing procedures and ongoing assessment to prevent site-specific or treatment-specific adverse events, such as pressure ulcers, thromboembolism or deep vein thrombosis, allergic reactions, or anticoagulation complications.

## Leapfrog Initiatives

Leapfrog is a consortium of healthcare purchasers/employers providing benefits to millions of Americans. The focus initially was on reducing healthcare costs by preventing medical errors and "leaping forward" by rewarding hospitals and healthcare organizations that improve safety and quality of care. Leapfrog has developed a number of initiatives to improve safety. These initiatives can be valuable tools in assessing and developing a patient safety culture. Leapfrog provides an annual Hospital Safety Grade and Hospital Survey to assess progress, release regional data, and encourage voluntary public reporting. **Initiatives investigated in the Leapfrog Hospital Survey** include:

- Safer health care:
  - Hand hygiene programs and audits.
  - Nursing workforce.
  - Culture of safety.
  - Leadership focused on safety.
  - Teamwork training.
- Infection rates for nosocomial infections.
- Reduction of mortality in the ICU by focusing on ICU staffing.
- Implementing safe surgical volumes for high-risk surgeries.
- Implementing hospital-wide never event policies.
- Using bar code technology to reduce medication errors.

This data is then compiled for tracking risk and improvement measures.

## Agency for Healthcare Research and Quality (AHRQ)

One tool to use in beginning an assessment of the healthcare organization's patient safety culture is a survey. The Agency for Healthcare Research and Quality (AHRQ) has sponsored the development of surveys for assessment of patient safety for different healthcare organizations, including hospitals, nursing homes, and outpatient facilities. These surveys are available for download and can be used easily for surveys of all levels of staff within an organization. The survey asks questions related to safety, error in medications/treatments, and incident reporting and typically take ≤15 minutes to complete, so they could be done as part of staff meetings or during clinical hours. The survey comprises questions about a number of sections, utilizing a scale of 1-5, checklists, and narrative for responses. Sections include:

- Work area/unit
- Supervisor/manager
- Communication
- Reporting patient safety events
- Patient safety rating
- Hospital/facility
- Background information
- Comments

## Failure Mode and Effects Analysis

Failure mode and effects analysis (FMEA) is a team-based prospective analysis method that attempts to identify and correct failures in a process before utilization to ensure positive outcomes. Steps in the process include:

1. Definition: Describe process and scope.
2. Team creation
3. Description: Flowchart with each step in the process numbered consecutively and substeps lettered consecutively.
4. Brainstorming each step for potential failure modes.
5. Identification of potential causes of failures: Root-cause analysis.
6. Listing potential adverse outcomes (to patients).
7. Assignment of severity rating: Adverse outcomes rated on a 1-10 scale for severity of failure.
8. Assignment of frequency/occurrence rating: Potential failures rated on a 1-10 scale for probability of failure in the prescribed time period.
9. Assignment of detection rating: Potential failures rated on a 1-10 scale for the probability that they will be identified before their occurrence.
10. Calculation of risk priority number (RPN): severity occurrence, and detection ($S \times O \times D$) to find the RPN.
11. Reduction of potential failures: Brainstorming.
12. Identification of performance measures.

## Root Cause Analysis

Root cause analysis (RCA) provides information about causes of adverse or sentinel events, but analysis requires careful review to determine if the RCA was done correctly. In many cases, an adverse event is the result of a series of errors or system problems rather than one clearly identifiable process failure. Environmental factors, such as staff reduction and poor floor design, can affect outcomes, as can poor communication, so factors that contribute in some way to the event (fatigue, poor design, inexperienced staff) but are not the direct cause must be identified in order to formulate action plans that will improve outcomes. Those reviewing the RCA must be objective, without bias that may influence their interpretation, such as assuming human error rather than systemic error is at fault, and must allow adequate time for decision making. In assessing the root cause, it is also important to consider how retrospective information available from the RCA may differ from information available to those involved in the procedure related to the sentinel/adverse event.

### *The Five Whys*

The 5 Whys is a method of finding root causes and solving problems that was designed by Taiichi Ohno, of Toyota, Japan. This process requires a team comprised of those who are knowledgeable about the process. Essentially, the team asks "why" in a sequential manner, usually at least five times, as an exercise to narrow the focus and arrive at a consensus about the cause of an event. Steps include:

- Outline the process in detail with each event ordered in the sequence of events described.
- Ask "why" questions about each step in the sequence of events to try to determine cause. For example:
  - Why did the patient return to the emergency department? Because the doctor failed initially to order an x-ray of the injured hand.

- Why did the doctor fail to order an x-ray of the injured hand? Because the x-ray department was understaffed and there was a 2-hour delay.

- Reach consensus and propose solutions to improve performance.

## *Is/Is Not*

Is/is not is a method to identify root causes and make decisions by determining what a problem/event is and what it is not. The purpose of is/is not is to keep the team focused on the immediate problem. Steps include creating a table with the problem at the top and columns for "is" and "is not" and filling in the table by doing the following:

- **Identify what the problem/event *is***: Ask what, why, when, where, how, and how much in relation to the process rather than focusing on the people involved. Create a detailed description of the problem/event.
- **Identify what the problem/event *is not***: Ask about which things could have caused the same problem but did not. Evaluate similar processes in which the problem did not occur.
- **Compare**: The two columns of information are examined to determine what distinguishes them, helping to find potential causes
- **Identify changes**: Note changes that may have occurred, resulting in the problem, leading to a root cause.

## Ishikawa "Fishbone" Diagram

The Ishikawa "fishbone" diagram, resembling the head and bones of a fish, is an analysis tool to determine causes and effects. In performance improvement, it is used to help identify root causes and make decisions. Typically, the "head" is labeled with the problem (the effect). Then, each bone is labeled with a category (causes), traditionally M (used for manufacturing), P (used for administration and service), and S (used for service):

- M: methods, materials, manpower, machines, measurement, Mother Nature (environment)
- P: people, process, prices, promotion, places, policies, procedures, product
- S: surroundings, suppliers, systems, skills

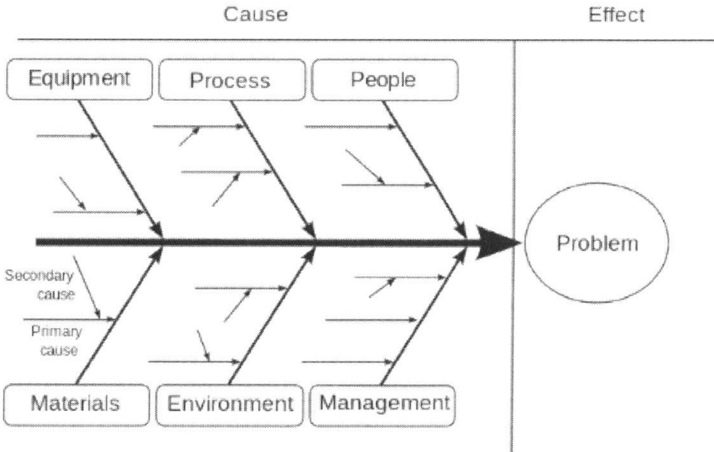


The categories serve only as a guide and can be selected and modified as needed. For example, if the effect is urinary tract infections, then all possible causes, derived from brainstorming, would be listed on the "bones": people, places, product, surroundings, material Then, each category listed would be questioned: "What are the issues affecting this category?" "What is the problem?" "Why is it happening?"

## Just Culture

While it is common practice to blame the individual responsible for committing an error, in a just culture, the practice is to look at the bigger picture and to try to determine what characteristics of the system are at fault, leading to the error. For example, there may be inadequate staffing, excessive overtime, unclear orders, mislabeling, or other problems that contribute. A just culture considers the need to change the system rather than the individual and differentiates among the following:

- **Human error**: Inadvertent actions, mistakes, or lapses in proper procedure. Management includes considering processes, procedures, training, and/or design to determine the cause of the error and consoling the person.
- **At-risk behavior**: Unjustified risk, choice. Management includes providing incentives for correct behavior and disincentives for incorrect, and coaching the person.
- **Reckless behavior**: Conscious disregard for proper procedures. Management includes remedial action and/or punitive action.

## Chain of Command

The Joint Commission has established leadership standards that apply to healthcare organizations and help to establish management's chain of command and accountability. Under these standards, leadership comprises the governing body, chief executive officer and senior managers, department leaders, leaders (both elected and appointed) of staff or departments, and the nurse executive and other nurse leaders. The governing body is ultimately responsible for all patient care rendered by all types of practitioners (physicians, nurses, laboratory staff, and support staff) within and under the jurisdiction of the organization, so this governing body must clearly outline the line of authority and accountability for others in management positions. At each level of management, performance standards and performance measurements should be established so that accountability becomes transparent based on data that can be used to drive changes when needed to bring about improved outcomes.

## Identifying and Responding to Gaps in Practice

### *Sentinel Events*

Sentinel events are defined by the Joint Commission as a death or serious physical injury that is unexpected. This death or injury could be related to many things, including surgery on the wrong body part, suicide, or infection. An infection is considered a sentinel event if it is determined that the death or injury would not have occurred without the infection. Each case must be dealt with individually, and, if defined as sentinel, a root cause analysis that defines the problem through gathering evidence to identify what contributed to the problem must be done. Once a root cause has been determined, an action plan that identifies all the different elements that contributed to the problem is recommended and instituted. The theory is that finding the root cause can eliminate the problem rather than just treating it. Thus, finding the source of an infection would be more important than just treating the infection.

### *Reportable Events and Never Events*

Each medical facility should have an established policy that identifies problems and **reportable events,** such as quality variances, sentinel events, and infections, which pose a risk to the quality of care and patient safety as well as data triggers that should prompt a case review or analysis. The policy should clearly define problems (such as sentinel events) and outline the processes for reporting, recording, and managing the problems, as well as appropriate preventive methods. Depending on the type of event, the nurse identifying a problem usually reports to the physician, supervisor, and other appropriate departments, such as the infection control officer, and/or regulatory agencies. Suicides are the second most common sentinel event reported to the Joint Commission. "**Never events,**" those that should never happen in a medical care setting, such as suicide, accidental death, or medication errors, should always be reported according to established procedures.

### AUDITS

An audit is a comprehensive systematic review to identify problems or gaps in practice. Types of audits include:

- **Culture**: The purpose of a culture audit at an organization is to assess the overall perceptions and values of an organization. The culture audit looks at the culture of the organization at all different levels. Culture audits may include surveys to ascertain how individuals feel about the organization, observations, focus groups, and review of documents. A culture audit should review the power structure of an organization and attitudes toward the power structure as well as the social structure.
- **Research**: The researcher should carefully document all decisions regarding the development of a program or research design (audit trail) to help eliminate as much personal bias as possible.
- **Efficiency**: The allocation of resources is analyzed to determine if they are allocated and used effectively, including both human and non-human resources. The audit may also evaluate compliance with laws and regulations.

#### PURPOSE OF PROGRAM AUDITS

The purpose of a program audit is to evaluate a program's performance to determine if the program is meeting its goals and performing effectively. The audit should be objective and independent. An audit action plan should be completed as part of the planning process to document the steps that will be taken during the audit. The program audit should review the program in relation to its mission, vision, goals, and outcomes. The program audit comprises a number of specialized audits. An efficiency audit is conducted to determine if resources are being managed effectively both in allocation and use while a financial audit looks at the budget in depth as well as reporting processes and all financial statements to determine if finances meet accounting standards. Another aspect of a program audit is the compliancy audit that evaluates regulatory compliance for state, federal, and accreditation regulations.

## Legal and Regulatory

### SENSITIVE INFORMATION

Sensitive information is classified under HIPAA as protected health information (PHI) and includes:

- Any information about an individual's past, present, or future health or condition (mental or physical)
- Provision of health care provided to the individual
- Any information related to payment for healthcare services that can be used to identify the person
- Identifying information: Name, address, Social Security number, birthdate, and any document or material that contains the identifying information (such as laboratory records)

Information that is to be shared or aggregated for research purposes must first be deidentified. The HIPAA privacy rule provides two methods of deidentification:

- Expert determination (based on applying statistical or scientific principles): The expert must have appropriate knowledge and must document the method and analysis results.
- Safe harbor (removing 18 types of identifiers): Includes names, geographic information, zip codes, telephone numbers, license numbers, account numbers, fax numbers, serial numbers of devices, email addresses, URLs, full-face photographs, dates (except year) and biometric identifiers

**Review Video: What is HIPAA**
Visit mometrix.com/academy and enter code: 412009

### *Protection of Organizational Sensitive Information*

When protecting sensitive information, the organization must first identify which information should be protected and where and how the information is stored and what type of safeguard is currently in place in order to ensure protection. Data stored in a single database may be easier to secure that those stored in separate databases. Data stored on paper, such as in files, or on individual computers can be easily lost and/or accessed. Examples of sensitive information include names and contact information (addresses, telephone numbers), characteristics (age, marital status, religion, gender), personally identifiable information (Social Security number, ID number, driving license number, mother's maiden name, credit/criminal history), financial data (credit cards, bank account numbers, PINs, security codes, health information, insurance information, and employment status). Once sensitive information is identified and located and vulnerabilities are determined, a comprehensive plan must be developed, based on review of data and processes, to protect information.

### *HIPAA Regulations for Sensitive Information Protection*

HIPAA mandates privacy and security rules (CFR, Title 45, part 164) to ensure that health information and individual privacy is protected:

- **Privacy rule**: Protected information includes any information included in the medical record (electronic or paper), conversations between the doctor and other healthcare providers, billing information, and any other form of health information. Procedures must be in place to limit access and disclosures.
- **Security rule**: Any electronic health information must be secure and protected against threats, hazards, or nonpermitted disclosures, in compliance with established standards. Implementation specifications must be addressed for any adopted standards. Administrative, physical, and technical safeguards must be in place as well as policies and procedures to comply with standards. Security requirements include: limiting access to those authorized, use of unique identifiers for each user, automatic logoff, encryption and decryption of protected healthcare information, authentication that healthcare data has not been altered/destroyed, monitoring of logins, authentication, and security of transmission. Access controls must include unique identifier, procedure to access system in emergencies, time out, and encryption/decryption.

### HIPAA's Protection of Privacy

As an integral member of the health care team, the nurse must always be aware of HIPAA regulations and apply this knowledge to practice. The nurse is responsible for the following efforts to protect and maintain patient privacy:

- The nurse must read and follow facility policies regarding the transfer of patient data.
- Communication between health care personnel about a patient should always be in a private place so that this information is not overheard by those who do not have the right to share the information.
- Access to charts must be restricted to only those health care team members involved in that patient's care.
- Patient care information for unlicensed workers cannot be posted at the bedside, but must be on a care plan or the patient chart in a protected area.
- The nurse must not give information casually to anyone (e.g., visitors or family members) unless it is confirmed that they have the right to have that information.
- Family members must not be relied upon to interpret for the patient; an interpreter must be obtained to protect patient privacy.
- Computers with patient information must have passwords and safeguards to prevent unauthorized access of patient information.
- The nurse should not leave voicemail messages containing protected healthcare information for a patient but should instead ask the patient to call back.

### HIPAA Breach Notification

HIPAA Breach Notification Rule requires covered entities to report any breaches in protected health information:

- **Individuals**: Notification by standard mail or email (if the individual has agreed) as soon as possible but no later than 60 days after the breach. If lacking contact information for 10 or more individuals, notice must be placed on the organization's website for 90 days with a tollfree telephone number or notice provided in print or broadcast media. For fewer than 10 individuals, alternate notification, such as by telephone, is permitted. Individual breaches are reported to the HHS Secretary annually.
- **500 or more individuals**: In addition to individual notification, notice must be given to a prominent media outlet serving the affected states no later than 60 days after the breach. The HHS Secretary must be notified electronically within 60 days after the breach. If the breach affected fewer than 500 individuals, the HHS Secretary must be notified within 60 days of the end of the calendar year in which the breaches occurred

## Copyright Law

### US Copyright Act

According to the US Copyright Act, as soon as an original work is fixed in any medium (print, photography, painting, video, audio, web page, illustration, dramatic works, computer software, architectural works, and music), it is automatically protected by copyright regardless of whether a copyright is applied for or stated. The work must be original and not copied and must involve some degree of creativity. While some work not in English may be in the public domain, a new translation of the work is copyrighted. Facts, such as dates and names, are not protected by copyright although a compilation of facts in an original manner is generally covered. Additionally, a photographic reproduction of a copyrighted work is not sufficiently original to qualify for copyright. Ideas are not protected, but words are. However, an oral presentation that is not recorded in any way is not covered by copyright. Works of the federal government, such as the CDC, are not copyrightable.

### *Fair Use Statute*

The Fair Use statute of the US Copyright Law allows for the use of copyrighted material without obtaining rights in limited circumstances, primarily in education and librarianship (but not for commercial purposes). The four issues that must be considered include:

- **Purpose of use**: Educational use may include photocopying articles, projecting images, or playing audio/visual recordings. Internet postings should be password protected so they have limited access. Transforming works, such as writing a parody, or using works for academic analysis are allowable.
- **Nature of the work**: Nonfiction work is more likely to be covered by fair use than fiction. Consumable works, such as workbook pages, are not considered appropriate for fair use.
- **Amount**: Generally, part of a work is fair use while the entire work may or may not be.
- **Effect**: The use should not compete in the market with the original. For example, copying and selling copies of the chapter of a book would compete with sales of the book.

## Zero Tolerance Policies

The trend in health care has moved away from the goal of maintaining adverse effects, such as bloodstream infections associated with central venous catheters, below national averages to zero tolerance. This requires a strong emphasis on preventive measures and best practices as well as continuing education and monitoring. All staff members must be educated about zero tolerance and best practices through classes, mentoring, posters, and self-study modules. Zero tolerance also applies to behavior, such as zero tolerance for drug diversion or negligence. All staff members must be informed of zero tolerance policies and have a clear understanding of actions that will be taken if zero tolerance policies are breached. The ANA has recently taken a zero-tolerance position on violence of any kind in the workplace, including not only acts of physical violence but also bullying and incivility. The ANA recommends providing a mechanism for support, informing employees of strategies for conflict resolution, and educating staff about bullying and prevention strategies

## Older Americans Act

The Older Americans Act (OAA) (Title III) of 1965 (amended in 2006 and reauthorized through fiscal year 2024) provides improved access to services for older adults and Native Americans, including community services (meals, transportation, home health care, adult day care, legal assistance, and home repair). The OAA provides funding to local **area agencies on aging (AAA)**, state, or tribal agencies, which administer funding. These local agencies can assess community needs and contract for services. One of the programs commonly supported with funds from the OAA is meals-on-wheels. Low-cost adult day care is also offered in some communities. The OAA includes the **National Family Caregivers Support Act**, which provides services for caregivers of older adults. The OAA also provides grants for programs that combat violence against older adults and others to provide computer training for older adults. Additionally, the OAA mandates that each state must have an ombudsman program. Ombudsmen provide services to residents of nursing homes and other facilities to ensure that care meets state standards.

## Americans with Disabilities Act

The 1990 Americans with Disabilities Act (ADA) is civil rights legislation that provides the disabled, including those with mental impairment, access to employment and the community. While employers must make reasonable accommodations for the **disabled**, the provisions related to the community apply more directly to **older Americans**. The ADA covers not only obvious disabilities but also disorders such as arthritis, seizure disorders, psychiatric disorders, cardiovascular, and respiratory disorders. Communities must provide transportation services for the disabled, including accommodation for wheelchairs. Public facilities (schools, museums, physician's offices, post offices, restaurants) must be accessible with ramps and elevators as needed. Telecommunications must also be accessible through devices or accommodations for the deaf and blind. **Compliance** is not yet complete because older buildings are required to provide access that is possible without "undue hardship," but newer construction of public facilities must meet ADA regulations.

## Occupational Safety and Health Administration (OSHA)

The **Occupational Safety and Health Act (OSHA)** seeks to keep workers safe and healthy while on the job. OSHA mandates that employers maintain a safe environment, workers are made fully aware of any hazards, and that access to personal protective gear is made available to workers who come into contact with hazardous materials. By following these regulations, an employer keeps injury and illness of workers to an absolute minimum. This fosters productivity, since workers are not absent due to illness or injury, employee health costs are contained, and the turnover rate is decreased, saving money spent on hiring and training new employees. OSHA is concerned about healthcare employee exposure to radiation, as well as chemical and biological agents, when caring for patients. Information is available to help hospitals and other facilities write plans that comply with best practices to deal with this and other threats to employees. Cleaning procedures, decontamination, and hazardous waste disposal are all covered by OSHA and apply to everyday hospital operation as well as disaster situations.

**Review Video: What is OSHA (Occupational Safety and Health Administration)**
Visit mometrix.com/academy and enter code: 913559

## Emergency Medical Treatment and Active Labor Act (EMTALA)

The Emergency Medical Treatment and Active Labor Act (EMTALA) is designed to prevent patient "dumping" from emergency departments (ED) and is an issue of concern for risk management that requires staff training for compliance:

- Transfers from the ED may be intrahospital or to another facility.
- Stabilization of the patient with emergency conditions or active labor must be done in the ED prior to transfer, and initial screening must be given prior to inquiring about insurance or ability to pay.
- Stabilization requires treatment for emergency conditions and reasonable belief that, although the emergency condition may not be completely resolved, the patient's condition will not deteriorate during transfer.
- Women in the ED in active labor should deliver both the child and placenta before transfer.
- The receiving department or facility should be capable of treating the patient and dealing with complications that might occur.
- Transfer to another facility is indicated if the patient requires specialized services not available intrahospital, such as to burn centers.

## FDA, Code of Federal Regulations, Title 21, Volume 1

The Food and Drug Administration, Code of Federal Regulations, Title 21, Volume 1 regulates protection of human subjects and states that any researcher using patients in research must obtain informed consent, in language understandable to the patient or the patient's agent. The elements of this informed consent must include an explanation of the research, the purpose, and the expected duration, as well as a description of any potential risks. Potential benefits and possible alternative treatments must be described. Any compensation to be provided must be outlined. The extent of confidentiality should be clarified. Contact information should be provided in the event the patient/family has questions. The patient must be informed that participation is voluntary and that he or she can discontinue participation at any time without penalty. Informed consent must be documented by a signed, written agreement. Principles of beneficence (maximize benefits and minimize harm) and justice (fair procedures and fair benefits) must be followed.

## Health and Human Services, Title 45 Code of Federal Regulations

Protection of human subjects is covered in the Health and Human Services, Title 45 Code of Federal Regulations, part 46. This provides guidance for institutional review boards (IRBs) for those involved in research and outlines requirements. Institutions engaged in nonexempt research must submit an assurance of compliance (document) to the Office of Human Research Protections (OHRP), agreeing to comply with all requirements for research projects. Subjects cannot be used solely as a means to an end; research should hold the possibility of benefit to the subject. Risks should be minimal, and selection of subjects should be equitable. Some research populations are granted additional protections because of their vulnerability and susceptibility to coercion; this includes children, prisoners, pregnant women, human fetuses and neonates, mentally disabled people, and people who are economically or educationally disadvantaged. When cooperative research projects are conducted involving more than one institution, then each must safeguard the rights of subjects, ensuring informed consent and privacy.

### *Institutional Review Boards*

An institutional review board (IRB) is a committee within an institution that is charged with reviewing research projects involving human subjects. The IRB reviews research proposals, approves them, monitors progress, and reviews outcomes. The IRB may conduct a risk-benefit analysis as part of an assessment to determine if the research is an advantage to the organization. The primary role of the IRB is to ensure that human subjects do not experience psychological or physical harm as the result of the research, that the research is carried out in an ethical manner, that regulatory guidelines are followed, and that subjects have informed consent and understand their rights. IRBs are regulated by the Office of Human Research Protections (OHRP), which is part of the US Department of Health and Human Services (HHS). The IRB is required to register with the OHRP and to obtain a Federalwide Assurance (FWA) before any research is carried out with federal funds.

## Genetic Information Nondiscrimination Act

The Genetic Information Nondiscrimination Act (2009) prohibits employers from using genetic information (genetic tests of the individual or individual's family members) to make decisions about employing individuals. This act is under the jurisdiction of the Equal Employment Opportunity Commission (EEOC). Covered entities (such as employers, employment agencies, labor-management training programs, and apprenticeship programs) cannot purchase or use genetic information in decision making. Information obtained indirectly, such as by overhearing comments, cannot be used as well. No genetic information can be used in employment decisions. This act also provides protection for the individual with a genetic disorder by prohibiting any type of harassment, such as making derogatory comments about the individual's disorder. DNA testing for law enforcement is allowed under the act, but the information can only be used for the legal proceedings. Covered entities must keep all genetic information confidential, regardless of how the information was obtained.

## HITECH Act

The American Recovery and Reinvestment Act (2009) (ARRA) included the **Health Information Technology for Economic and Clinical Health Act (HITECH),** which provided incentives for healthcare providers to switch to electronic health records and allowed patients greater access to their electronic health records. Security provisions include:

- Individuals and HHS must be notified of breach in security of personal health information.
- Business partners must meet security regulations or face penalties.
- The sale/marketing of personal health information is restricted.
- Individuals must have electronic access to electronic health information, although the law doesn't specify the form that the disclosed information must take (email, CD, web portal). Copies must be in a format that is readable if the individual requests it, and the healthcare provider may charge a fee.
- Individuals must be informed of disclosures of personal health information.
- Individual can direct healthcare providers to transmit a copy of their health records to individuals or entities of their choosing.

## National Healthcare Safety Network (NHSN)

The National Healthcare Safety Network (NHSN) integrates and replaces three separate programs: National Nosocomial Infections Surveillance (NNIS), Dialysis Surveillance Network (DSN), and National Surveillance System for Health Care Workers (NaSH). All healthcare facilities, such as hospitals and dialysis centers, can participate in the internet-based program that allows for reporting and sharing data. Those who apply to become members must agree to utilize CDC definitions, follow strict protocols, and submit data every six months. Anonymity of the institutions is protected. The program streamlines reporting of data and provides comparative data from across the United States. The system can identify sentinel or unusual events and notify appropriate participating agencies. There are three components to NHSN: patient safety, healthcare worker safety, and research and development. Extensive data analysis features are part of the program. Reports of nosocomial, or hospital-acquired, infections that were previously issued by NNIS are now issued by NHSN.

## Medicare

Medicare, a federally directed program, was introduced by the Title XIX Social Security Act in 1965. It provides health insurance to elderly patients and to patients with disabilities. The patient who is covered will receive hospital, doctor, and further medical care as needed. The patient's income is not a factor for eligibility. **Original Medicare** consists of **Part A** and **Part B**, and covers the majority of medical care when the patient seeks care at a facility that accepts Medicare. If the patient requires prescription drug assistance, they may opt into **Part D**, which is the Medicare drug plan, or they may opt into the **Medicare Advantage Plan (Part C),** which bundles Parts A, B and D.

### *Medicare Part A*

Medicare Part A covers hospital care (inpatient), care at a skilled nursing facility or nursing home, hospice care, and home health care. Anyone 65 years of age or older that is eligible to receive **Social Security** is automatically enrolled even if still working. Patients are also able to receive Social Security if they or their spouse put money into the system by way of working for at least 40 quarters. If the patient has less than 40 quarters of work, Medicare Part A requires a payment each month. If the patient is not yet 65 but has a complete disability that will remain for the rest of their life, Medicare Part A can be used after receiving Social Security benefits for 2 years. A patient with ongoing renal disease who needs either dialysis or transplant can become eligible for Part A without waiting for 2 years.

### Medicare Part B

Medicare Part B covers both medically necessary services and preventive services such as doctor visits, physical therapy, occupational therapy, speech therapy, medical equipment, assessments, clinical research, mental health support and wellness visits. The patient has to **pay a monthly premium for Medicare Part B,** which is either directly billed to the patient or deducted from their Social Security or other benefit payment. The program covers 80% of the authorized expense for any medical attention that is required (following a yearly deductible).

## Medicaid

1965 Title XIX Social Security Act introduced **Medicaid** as a federal/state matching plan for low-income individuals supervised by the federal government. Funding comes from federal and state taxes, with no less than 50%, but no more than 83% being funded federally. Each state is able to add optional eligibility criteria on the list, and they may also put restrictions (to a point) on federally directed aid. Patients who receive Medicaid cannot get a bill for the aid, but states are able to require small copayments or deductibles for particular types of help.

Federal regulations require that states support certain individuals or groups of individuals through Medicaid, although not everyone who falls below the federal poverty rate is eligible. **Mandatory eligibility groups** include the following:

- Patients deemed categorically needy by their state, and receive financial support from various federal assistance programs.
- Individuals receiving Federal Supplemental Security income (SSI).
- Patients that are older than 65 that are blind or have complete disability.
- Pregnant women and children younger than 6 years of age who live in families that are up to 133% of the federal poverty level (some states allow for a higher income to meet eligibility in this class).
- Adults under the age of 65 that make less than or equal to 133% of the federal poverty level and are not receiving Medicare.

**Review Video: Medicare & Medicaid**
Visit mometrix.com/academy and enter code: 507454

## Integrating Legal, Regulatory, and Documentation Requirements

Legal and regulatory requirements should be integrated into all nursing professional development activities because the provision of medical care is increasingly governed by state, federal, and accreditation regulations and requirements. Healthcare organizations must meet regulatory standards for reimbursement from Medicare and Medicaid. Accreditation agencies, such as the Joint Commission, have had a profound influence on performance standards. Nursing personnel must stay abreast of changes in standards associated with the primary regulatory and accrediting agencies and should have a clear understanding of how these standards relate to quality outcomes. Healthcare providers at all levels must be updated when changes occur, and processes and practices may need to be changed. Documentation requirements may also change, and failure to understand new requirements may adversely affect reimbursement. Additionally, since the Joint Commission now conducts unannounced surveys, nursing staff must be aware of and constantly compliant with accreditation standards.

# Evidence-Based Practice and Research

## Research Process

### Research and Scholarship

The professional development nurse has a responsibility to be involved in research and scholarship. Research must be planned and carried out with standard research methods. All nurses are expected to research and apply evidence-based practices to nursing care. Clinical research may be based on observation of patients' needs or lack of adequate research findings or conflicting findings regarding an issue, and may involve collaboration with an interdisciplinary group of healthcare providers. Scholarship involves not only continuing formal education to an advanced degree but also sharing information gleaned from research, such as through publications of articles in journals and/or books, presentations at conferences, and authoring continuing-education courses. Professional development nurses may also develop posters, handouts, videos, and slide shows as part of scholarship activities. Additionally, professional development nurses may serve as instructors in nursing programs and mentors and/or preceptors to nursing students.

### Tracking and Trending to Identify Problems

Tracking and trending is central to developing research-supported evidence-based practice and is part of continuous quality improvement as it helps to identify problems. Once processes and outcomes measurements are selected, at least one measure should be tracked for a number of periods of time, usually in increments of 4 weeks or quarterly. This tracking can be used to present graphical representation of results that will show trends. While trends will show some normal variation, if the trend becomes erratic and measures are inconsistent, this suggests that the processes of care are not consistent or are inadequate. For example, if infections in PICC lines are tracked and the trend shows wild fluctuations with high levels of infection in one period, low in another, and vacillations in a third, then the first step is to ensure that the process is being followed correctly. If the process is stable but the variations persist, then the next course would be to modify the process by looking at best practices.

### Steps to the Research Process

Steps to the research process are as follows:

1. Identify a problem: Focus first on a broad topic and then narrow it to a specific question.
2. Conduct literature review: Review existing research on the topic, including meta-analyses.
3. Develop theoretical framework: Choose a feasible method of reaching a solution to the problem.
4. Develop hypothesis: Select a hypothesis that predicts expected outcomes.
5. Identify a research design: Identify the design as experimental (researcher introduces an intervention) or nonexperimental (researcher collects data).
6. Specify population: Specify type, number, and characteristics of population.
7. Manage variables: Devise methods to identify and measure variables.
8. Conduct pilot study: Conduct a small-scale study of the major project to improve the project.
9. Select sample: Use care in selecting a representative sample, using sampling procedures.
10. Collect data: Train staff to collect data, keeping accurate records.
11. Prepare and analyze data: Organize data and conduct both qualitative and quantitative analysis of data.
12. Interpret and communicate results: Critically evaluate findings and prepare research report.

## Research Results

Analysis of data and outcomes is the basis for research results, which may be categorized as follows:

- **Significant/Predicted (Positive):** These results are those expected by the researcher and generally support the logic of the study, although alternative reasons for the results should be explored.
- **Non-significant (Negative):** These results indicate that the hypothesis is in error, although an inadequate sample or weak methodology may obscure significance.
- **Significant/Non-predicted**: These results are opposite of those expected but may add to knowledge about the subject. Researcher bias may lead some researchers to disregard results that they do not anticipate.
- **Mixed**: These results are the most common with different variables yielding different results. Methodology or theory may need modification.
- **Unexpected**: These results, also referred to as serendipitous, are completely unpredicted and a different study may be needed to examine their significance.

## Research Designs

### *Descriptive Research*

Descriptive research is intended to explore and describe people, events, or groups in real-life situations in order to develop new information or knowledge about the subjects. Descriptive research is especially useful when researching a subject about which there is little information so that the researchers understand how situations naturally occur. An example would be a study looking at the symptoms of survivors of disasters and the variables that affect outcomes. The design begins by identifying a phenomenon of interest and then selecting a number of variables that may influence the phenomenon. A descriptive research project does not involve intervention or treatment but rather observation. The variables are described and measured. Different methods may be employed, including direct observation, measurements, and questionnaires to obtain information. Descriptive designs may be comparative, examining the differences in variable between two or more groups, and time-dimensional, examining changes or trends over time.

### *Correlational Research*

Correlational research is intended to predict, test, or describe the relationships among different variables. A representative sample must be selected and the type and strength of the relationship examined rather than differences. Designs vary depending on the purpose. A descriptive correlational model that examines the relationship among variables may be utilized to develop a hypothesis. Predictive designs attempt to determine the effect that independent variables have on a dependent variable in order to predict a causal relationship. In a model-testing correlational design, a concept map is created that identifies all exogenous, endogenous, and residual variables. The three possible correlational outcomes of correlational research include:

- **Positive**: Variables increase or decrease simultaneously. Correlation coefficient is close to +1.
- **Negative**: If one variable increases, the other decreases, and vice versa. Correlation coefficient is close to -1.
- **None**: No correlation exists among variables. Correlation coefficient is close to 0.

#### *Quasi-Experimental Research*

Quasi-experimental research is a form of quantitative research intended to examine relationships and to determine the reason that events happen, examining the causal relationship between selected independent and dependent variables. Quasi-experimental designs are often used when complete control is impossible. Quasi-experimental research lacks random assignment but is otherwise similar to experimental studies in design. One common design is nonequivalent groups in which two nonrandomized groups are selected and exposed to different variables (such as two classrooms with different teaching approaches). Another design is regression-discontinuity. With this design, groups are divided according to predetermined criterion, such as a cutoff score on a test as a requirement for an intervention. Pre-test and post-test design involves identifying a group and administering a pre-test and then providing an intervention, followed by a post-test to determine the efficacy of the intervention.

#### *Experimental Research*

Experimental research provides the best control because it eliminates or controls factors that influence the dependent variable in order to determine causality. The primary elements of experimental research are randomization, manipulation of the independent variables by the research, and control of the experimental situation. There are many design models, but the classic experimental research design involves two randomized groups—one the experimental group and the other the control group. Both groups take a pre-test and then the experimental group undergoes an intervention of some type, and then both groups take a post-test to determine if the intervention had an effect. Another model uses only a post-test. The randomized blocking design follows the classic or post-test only design but involves blocking a variable that may interfere with results. That is, identifying the variable and assigning those with the variable according to severity or other ranking randomly to both groups so that the variable is balanced.

### Linking Evidence to Desired Outcomes

Linking evidence to desired outcomes requires careful planning. First, the desired outcomes must be identified and prioritized. Then, research projects that accomplished similar outcomes must be reviewed to determine if they are applicable. Issues to consider include the target population studied and how closely it aligns with the current population because, if it does not, the results of the same intervention may be quite different. Additionally, the methodology must be assessed to determine if it could be replicated. Whether or not the research has external validity is especially important. For example, research conducted at a small rural hospital may yield different outcomes from one conducted at a large urban hospital. If an intervention, based on evidence-based research, is implemented, then careful assessment must be done to determine if the intervention directly affected the outcomes or if other variables intervened

## Literature Review and Data Collection/Interpretation

### Literature Reviews

#### *Boolean Search*

Literature research requires comprehensive evaluation of current (no more than 5 years old) and/or historical information. Most literature research begins with an internet search of databases, which provide listings of books, journals, and other materials on specific topics. Databases vary in content and many contain only a reference listing with or without an abstract, so once the listing is obtained, the researcher must do a further search (publisher, library, etc.) to locate the material. Some databases require subscription, but access is often available through educational or healthcare institutions. In order to search effectively, the researcher should begin by writing a brief explanation of the research to help identify possible keywords and synonyms to use as search words:

- Truncations: "Finan*" provides all words that begin with those letters, such as "finance," "financial," and "financed."
- Wildcards: "m?n" or "m*n" provides "man" and "men"
- BOOLEAN logic (AND, OR, NOT):
- Wound OR infect* OR ulcer
- Wound OR ulcer AND povidone-iodine
- Wound AND povidone-iodine NOT antibiotic NOT antimicrobial

### SQL Search

Structured query language (SQL) is a fourth-generation programming language (4GL) that differs from 3GLs, such as Java, in that SQL uses syntax similar to human language to access, manipulate, and retrieve data from relational database management systems (RDBMS), which stores data in tables. Both the American National Standards Institute (ANSI) and the International Organization for Standardization (ISO) have adopted SQL as a standard; however, because the language is complex, many vendors do not utilize the complete standard, and this limits portability between vendors without modifications. Despite many available versions, ANSI standards require that basic commands (UPDATE, DELETE, SELECT, etc.) be supported. Language elements of SQL include:

- **Clauses**: From, where, group by, having, and order by
- **Expressions**: Produce scales and tables
- **Predicates**: 3-valued logic (null, true, false) and Boolean truth values
- **Queries**: The most commonly used SQL operation, require a SELECT statement
- **Statements**: Includes the semicolon (to terminate a statement)

### PICOT

The PICOT format is one method of developing appropriate questions to use in searching quantitative research. This method helps clarify the question and necessary information and to identify key words utilized in searching.

| | | |
|---|---|---|
| **P** | Patient/ Population | List important characteristics: 35-year-old male with low back pain |
| **I** | Intervention/ Indicator | Explain the desired intervention under consideration: Acupuncture |
| **C** | Comparison/ Control | List other possible interventions or alternatives: Surgery |
| **O** | Outcome | Provide the desired measurable outcomes: Decreased pain levels (from 6–7 to 1–2) and increased mobility |
| **T** | Time | Timeframe (if appropriate) |

This format is then used to formulate a question:

*In a 35-year-old male with low back pain, how does acupuncture compared with surgery affect pain levels and mobility?*

Based on this question, then the search may be conducted with the following (including synonyms): (back pain or sciatica) and (acupuncture or surgery) and (pain management or pain-free or pain control).

## Data Collection and Interpretation

### *Qualitative and Quantitative Data*

Both qualitative and quantitative data are used for analysis, but the focus is quite different:

- **Qualitative data**: Data are described verbally or graphically, and the results are subjective, depending upon observers to provide information. Interviews may be used as a tool to gather information, and the researcher's interpretation of data is important. Gathering this type of data can be time-intensive, and it can usually not be generalized to a larger population. This type of information gathering is often useful at the beginning of the design process for data collection.
- **Quantitative data**: Data are described in terms of numbers within a statistical format. This type of information gathering is done after the design of data collection is outlined, usually in later stages. Tools may include surveys, questionnaires, or other methods of obtaining numerical data. The researcher's role is objective.

### *Data Collection Methods for Qualitative Research*

Researchers engaged in qualitative research may need to use a variety of different collection methods, but it is important to determine how each collection strategy meets the needs of the study. Researchers need to determine who will collect the data and the methods that they will use. Data collection may include direct observations, surveys, interviews, and various other sources of information, such as documents and audiovisual materials. Field workers should be carefully trained so that there is consistency in their approaches to data collection to ensure that the data generated is meaningful. Storing data should always be a consideration as large studies may generate much data. There should be an organized method of storage for hard copies, such as field notes, as well as a computer software program that allows for various types of displays of the data to facilitate analysis.

# Evidence-Based Practice Process

## Institute of Healthcare Improvement

The Institute of Healthcare Improvement (IHI) is a nonprofit organization that promotes better and more cost-effective patient care with the goals of preventing needless deaths, pain and suffering, helplessness, excessive waiting, waste, and lack of care. IHI encourages such measures as the use of rapid response teams and medication reconciliation. IHI has developed bundles, a group of processes based on evidence-based practices that must be carried out in order to improve patient outcomes. Bundles include 3-5 steps, but each step is critical, and all steps should be performed as prescribed, as in the following examples for sepsis (first hour) and central line infection prevention:

| Sepsis Hour-1 Management | Central Line Infection Prevention |
|---|---|
| Measure lactate (and remeasure if level is >2 mmol/L).<br>Collect blood cultures prior to antibiotic administration.<br>Administer broad-spectrum antibiotics.<br>For hypotension or lactate >4 mmol/L: Rapid administration of crystalloid fluids (30 mL/kg).<br>If hypotension continues, initiate vasopressors for MAP goal > 65 mmHg. | Proper hand hygiene.<br>Use of barrier precautions (PPE).<br>Skin antisepsis with chlorhexidine.<br>Choosing the optimal site for catheter insertion.<br>Daily evaluation of catheter and assessment for potential removal. |

## Disease-Specific Certifications

In order to qualify for disease-specific care (DSC) certification under the Joint Commission, programs must meet general requirements for certification as well as specific requirements associated with the disease-specific domain. DSC programs include: acute stroke ready hospital, chronic kidney disease, COPD, comprehensive stroke center, heart failure, inpatient diabetes, lung-volume reduction surgery, palliative care, perinatal care, primary stroke center, total knee and total hip replacement, and ventricular assist device. As part of certification, the Joint Commission conducts an onsite review to determine how the organization uses outcomes and performance measures to improve care, whether the organization is committed to improving care, and how patients are educated and prepared for discharge. The reviewers evaluate the evidence-based guidelines in use and may utilize tracer methodology. Certification is granted for a 2-year period with a 1-year intracycle monitoring conference call. The Joint Commission utilizes the Survey Analysis for Evaluating Risk (SAFER) scoring methodology to evaluate risk of deficiencies.

## Best Available Evidence and Best Practices

Evidence-based research is the use of current research and individual values in practice to establish a plan of care for each individual. Research may be the result of large studies of best practices or individual research from observations in practice about the effectiveness of treatment. Evidence-based practice requires a commitment to ongoing research and outcomes evaluations. Many resources are available:

- Guide to Clinical Preventive Services by the Agency for Healthcare Research and Quality of the US Department of Health and Human Services

Evidence-based practice requires a thorough understanding of research methods in order to evaluate the results and determine if they can be generalized. Results must also be evaluated in terms of cost-effectiveness. Steps to evidence-based practice include:

1. Making a diagnosis
2. Researching and analyzing results
3. Applying research findings to plan of care
4. Evaluating outcomes

## Levels of Evidence

Levels of evidence are categorized according to the scientific evidence available to support the recommendations, as well as existing state and federal laws. While recommendations are voluntary, they are often used as a basis for state and federal regulations.

- **Category IA** is well supported by evidence from experimental, clinical, or epidemiologic studies and is strongly recommended for implementation.
- **Category IB** has supporting evidence from some studies, has a good theoretical basis, and is strongly recommended for implementation.
- **Category IC** is required by state or federal regulations or is an industry standard.
- **Category II** is supported by suggestive clinical or epidemiologic studies, has a theoretical basis, and is suggested for implementation.
- **Category III** is supported by descriptive studies, such as comparisons, correlations, and case studies, and may be useful.
- **Category IV** is obtained from expert opinion or authorities only.
- **Unresolved** means there is no recommendation because of a lack of consensus or evidence.

## Disseminating Findings

### *Types of Presentations/Meetings*

Methods of disseminating research and evidence-based practice findings include:

- **Oral/Podium presentations**: These are usually formal presentations based on a prepared outline and presented at conferences or other professional gathering. Oral/Podium presentations often involve the use of presentation software.
- **Panel discussions**: This allows for discussion of various approaches so the pros and cons can be discussed. Remarks may be prepared in advance in some situations.
- **Roundtable discussions**: These presentations are usually informal and include 6-12 participants. Usually up to a half of the time is spent in discussion, so presentation time is limited.
- **Small group/Team/Committee meetings**: Evidence-based practice findings may be disseminated during grand rounds and clinical rounds as well as at team meetings. Presentations to committee meetings are usually more formal.
- **Community meetings**: Presentations must be sensitive to cultural issues and consider different levels of health literacy. Presentations should be planned with community members.
- **Visual arts**: Information may be displayed in the form of posters and illustrations in print as well as online.
- **Vodcasts**: Information may be shared through vodcasts with limited or open access (such as on YouTube). Vodcasts should be carefully planned and scripted to ensure information is presented effectively. Vodcasts require knowledge of technology and are most likely to maintain attention if limited to about 15 minutes.
- **Audio/Podcasts**: These can be accessed at any time, so they are convenient but also require knowledge of technology. Podcasts should be limited to about 10 minutes to maintain interest.
- **Journal clubs: These may be virtual or on-site** and are usually led by a clinician with expertise in the area of study.
- **Publishing**: Journal articles (print and online) are one of the most effective means of disseminating findings to professionals.
- **Media**: It is important to consider the audience and their interests. Contacting the media may take time and requires preparation.

## Implementing Evidence-Based Practice

### *Engaging Stakeholders*

Engaging stakeholders, those with a vested interested in evidence-based practice, is critical to implementation. Stakeholders may include:

- Patients and their families, caregivers, and advocates: Information should be tied to personal interests so people understand benefits and presented in a manner that is understandable to the lay person, avoiding medical jargon or complex data.
- Healthcare providers: Clinicians need clear evidence of benefit to themselves and patients with supporting data.
- Healthcare organizations and associations: Emphasis should include benefits to the organization in terms of reduced error or improved patient care as well as cost-effectiveness and return-on-investment.

- Employers and insurers: The explanation for the need of coverage for any changes in practice should be clearly outlined, including data regarding benefits, such as reduced hospital stay or reduced complications.
- Health care industry/manufacturers: These may have product information that can be very helpful as part of implementation.
- Policymakers: Providing the most up-to-date information in a format that is easy to understand and supported by adequate data can help with decision making.

### *Models for Implementing Evidence-Based Practice*

A number of different models are used for implementing evidence-based practice:

- **Iowa Model**: Clinicians identify problem-focused and knowledge-focused triggers (practice questions) and consider whether they are priorities. They then form a team, assemble relevant research, critique and synthesize the research, determine efficacy of change, and pilot the change, followed by evaluating outcomes and determining if the change should be adopted. If so, results are disseminated.
- **Model for Evidence-Based Practice Change**: This 6-step cyclical process begins with assessing the need for change, collecting the best internal and external evidence, analyzing the evidence (weigh and synthesize), designing practice change and identifying resources, implementing and evaluating the practice change beginning with a pilot study, and integrating and maintaining the practice change by communicating with stakeholders, monitoring, and disseminating results.
- **John Hopkins Model**: Three major components include (1) practice question, (2) evidence, and (3) translation.
- **Stetler Model:** This practitioner-oriented model includes five steps: Preparation (research), validation (evaluate evidence), comparative evaluation/decision making (determine feasibility), translation/application (confirm and implement), and evaluation.
- **ARCC (Advancing Research and Clinical Practice through close Collaboration) Model for System-Wide Implementation and Sustainability of Evidence-Based Practice**: This model utilizes cognitive behavioral therapy to guide clinicians toward adopting evidence-based practice (EBP) by changing beliefs about EBP. Implementation begins by assessing organizational culture and readiness for change. Key strengths and weaknesses are identified. Questions are asked and research conducted. The EBP Beliefs Scale is used to assess practitioners' ability to implement changes.
- **Promoting Action on Research Implementation in Health Services Framework (PARIHS framework):** Elements include evidence (research, clinical and patient experience, and local data), context (the environment or setting for change, the culture of the organization), and facilitation (process of facilitating implementation, purpose, role, skills, and attributes). Elements have low (negative) and high (positive) subelements.
- **Clinical Scholar Model**: Based on information provided in 6-8 all-day workshops that focuses on educating, processing, and mentoring. Participants learn how to ask questions, research, and analyze research to bring about synthesis.

### *Barriers*

Barriers to implementing evidence-based practice may occur at the individual level as well as the organizational level. Individuals may lack the skills needed to research or to evaluate research even if they have an interest in change. Some individuals lack the motivation or confidence to promote change in practice, and others lack contact with other professionals who share their interests. Some individuals are comfortable with the way they have always done things and are reluctant to change even when faced with evidence. The most critical barriers, however, exist at the organizational level because making evidence-based changes can be both expensive and complex with many different factors to consider. Organizations may lack motivation to change and may be resistive to any increased costs. Leadership may be poor or inadequate; and, without the support of leadership, very little can be accomplished.

# Technology

## Information Systems and Management

### Information Management

#### *Policies*

Policies must be based on best practices and conform to state, federal, and accreditation regulations and guidelines. Empowerment includes encouraging participation of all staff in policy making. Objectives for policies should be clearly outlined. In some cases, policies may be broad and cover all aspects of an organization, but in other cases, policies may be much more specific, such as a policy regarding use of computer equipment. Conflict of interest policies should be in place to ensure that those involved in review activities should not be primary caregivers or have an economic or personal interest in a case under review. Policies should ensure that access to protected health information be limited to those who need the information to complete duties related to direct care or performance improvement review activities. Policy and procedure manuals should be readily available organization-wide in easily accessible format, such as online. Policy issues may include cost-effectiveness, insurance coverage, criteria for qualified staff, and legal implications.

#### *Physical Security*

Physical security is essential for computer systems. The first step is to determine who should have access to different types of equipment and then to apply methods to limit access to those authorized through use of user names and passwords/tokens. Servers should be maintained in locked, climate-controlled rooms with the servers mounted on racks and under surveillance. Vulnerable devices should remain in the locked room. Data should be backed up routinely and stored/archived in a secure remote location. Workstations should be secure, including printers. Cable lock systems should be used to secure equipment, including laptops, to furniture. Operating systems should be locked when not in use and encryption software used to secure routers used for wireless transmission. Equipment should be in restricted areas. Remote access should be done with secure modems and encryption. Public access to the internet should be on a different network from that used to transmit healthcare information.

#### *Access and Passwords*

Passwords, which are usually used with a username and are used to access protected data, should be changed every 30-60 days. More frequent changes make it hard for people to remember their passwords, so they are more likely to write them down, increasing the risk of security breaches. Strong passwords include combinations of letters (capital and lower case), numbers, and symbols/signs, such as the ampersand (&), and are harder to break than dictionary words. Users should never share passwords.

Tokens are items used to authenticate a person's identity and allow access to a system. They commonly require the use of not only the token but also a PIN or user name and password. Tokens may be in the form of access cards, which may utilize different technologies: photos, optical-coding, electric circuits, and magnetic strips. They may also be contained in common objects, such as a key fob. Some tokens must be plugged directly into the computer. Different types of tokens include: ID cards, challenge-response tokens, and smart cards.

## Information Systems

### Databases

Databases are computerized file structures that contain organized and accessible stored data. Hierarchical databases, the earliest type, are organized in a tree or parent-child formation with one piece of information connected to many (one-to-many), but in descending order only (not many-to-one). Hierarchical databases are appropriate only for simple structures (such as lists of email addresses or telephone numbers) and have limited use in health care. Hierarchical databases have largely been replaced with relational databases, which are built on a multiple table structure with each individual item on a table having a unique identifier. The tables (or relationships) can be manipulated. Each table represents an item or thing. Tables are comprised of rows (records, which must be unique) and columns (fields). Relational databases allow both one-to-many and many-to-one relationships. Relational databases may contain >1000 tables, but through querying, new tables using the relationships among existing data can be produced.

### Cochrane Library

The Cochrane Library is a primary resource in the development of evidence-based practice. Cochrane provides a collection of different medical databases in the Cochrane Library for easy internet access. Cochrane databases include:

- Cochrane Database of Systemic Reviews
- Cochrane Methodology Register
- Health Technology Assessment (HTA) Database
- Database of Abstracts of Reviews of Effects (DARE)
- Cochrane Central Register of Controlled Trials (CENTRAL)
- NHS Economic Evaluation Database (NHS EED)

Cochrane also provides reviews of research and meta-analysis to synthesize the research findings of various research studies. Researchers for Cochrane conduct statistical analysis when comparing data from a variety of studies or trials. The Cochrane Library is freely accessed in many countries but requires a subscription for complete access to reports in US states. Other databases include the following: PubMed provides abstracts, the Cumulated Index of Nursing and Allied Health Literature (CINAHL) (owned by EBSCOhost) provides four databases, and Medscape Reference (part of WebMD) provides articles on many topics.

### Wikis

Wikis are websites or document collections (essentially databases) that are open-ended forums that allow users to add content or edit content that is already there. *Wikipedia* is one example. This type of learning community allows various users to collaborate on projects; however, there may be issues with copyright and factual accuracy with wikis, especially if participation is open to all. Wikis are particularly useful for group projects in which a limited access wiki is set up so that group members can easily collaborate on writing. Group members can view documents while engaging in a conference call rather than meeting in person. Because wikis are internet based, users can access a wiki with any internet connection from any place at any time. Instructors as well as learners can use wikis to collaborate.

### Learning Management Systems

Learning management systems (LMSs) are software applications that are used to present electronic educational material. Learning management systems not only provide content but also track students' progress, including participation and scores on quizzes and tests. Students may upload assignments, such as research papers. Learning management systems vary widely. Some simply manage training or course records while others provide a full suite of options for presenting and tracking online classes. The LMS alone is not used to create course content, but another software application that is often used in conjunction with the LMS is the learning content management system (LCMS), which allows the user to create course content that is stored in a central server so that the information and lessons can be used for other courses as well. Some LMSs allow for both synchronous and asynchronous use.

### ELECTRONIC HEALTH RECORDS

The electronic health record (EHR) is a digital computerized patient record that may be integrated with CPOE and CDSS to improve patient care and reduce medical error. Software applications vary considerably, and standardization has not yet been implemented, so the organization must carefully review current and future anticipated needs as well as the ability of applications to interface with each other to provide for adequate measurements, data collection, reports, retrieval of data, analysis, and confidentiality. Increasingly, physicians in private practice, especially those in large groups, are employing EMRs, which may be different systems than those used in hospitals. Systems can be customized to meet the needs of the organization, but cost and lack of standardization remain barriers for implementation. However, studies indicate that there is a positive correlation between comprehensive EMR systems and patient outcomes. Quantifiable data about cost-effectiveness can be difficult to calculate because savings are often in terms of saved time, fewer interventions, and reduced error.

## CPOE

Computerized physician/provider order entry (CPOE) programs are clinical software applications that automate medication/treatment ordering, requiring that orders be typed in a standard format to avoid mistakes in ordering or interpreting orders. CPOE is promoted by Leapfrog as a means to reduce medication errors. About 50% of medication errors occur during ordering, so reducing this number can have a large impact on patient safety. Most CPOE systems contain a clinical decision support system (CDDS) as well so that the system can provide an immediate alert related to patient allergies, drug interactions, duplicate orders, or incorrect dosing at the time of data entry. Some systems can also provide suggestions for alternative medications, treatments, and diagnostic procedures. The CPOE system may be integrated into the information system of the organization for easier tracking of information and data collection. This system is cost-effective, replaces handwritten orders, and allows easy access to patient records.

## CDSS

Clinical decision support systems (CDSS) are intended for the end user and comprise interactive software applications that provide information to physicians or other healthcare providers to help with healthcare decisions. The programs contain a base of medical knowledge to which patient data can be entered so an evidence-based inference system can provide patient specific advice. For example, a CDSS may be used in the emergency department so that staff can enter symptoms into the program and, based on the information entered, the CDSS program provides possible diagnoses and treatment options. The CDSS system may be used for a variety of purposes:

- Record keeping and documentation, such as authorization
- Monitoring of patient's treatments, research protocols, orders, and referrals
- Ensuring cost-effectiveness by monitoring orders to prevent duplication or tests that are not indicated by condition/symptoms
- Providing support in physician diagnosis and ensuring treatments are based on best practices

## Business Tools

### Email

Email is a valuable means of communication between learner and instructor, but the nursing professional development specialist should set clear boundaries and ensure that emails are secure. Email attachments should not be opened unless the receiver knows the sender and expects the attachment. Even running a virus scan program is not sufficient because new viruses may be undetectable. The most common method for uploading malicious coding or viruses to a computer or network is to send them through email as an attachment. For this reason, some organizations prohibit the use of email or prohibit opening of any attachments. When a perpetrator attempts to obtain another person's personal information, such as user name and password, through email by pretending to be an authorized individual, this is an example of phishing. Phishing emails may contain infected downloads or links to malware. The emails may contain links to fake websites that are replicas of the real websites. In some cases, phishing may involve instant messaging or pop-up windows that ask for verifying data.

### Document Production

A number of issues should be considered in document production:

- **Typography**: Typeface may be serif (especially print documents) or sans serif (more common online). Serif typefaces have small strokes at the end of letters. Serif typeface may appear blurry in online documents. Different typeface may be used for headings, but generally no more than three different typefaces should be used in a document.
- **Budget**: Costs for production, copying, distributing must be considered.
- **Timing**: Production should be planned according to the date the document is needed.
- **Access structure**: Headings and subheadings and content lists should be designed.
- **Numbering/Headers and footers/Page breaks**: Decisions include the type of numbering and whether to include heaters or footers. Decisions must be made regarding page breaks.
- **Text alignment/Margins**: Choices include justified, ranged right or left, centered.
- **Paragraphing**: Most single-spaced documents are left aligned with extra space between paragraphs while double-spaced documents have indented paragraphs.
- **Illustrations/Tables/Charts**: Size and alignment in the text must be determined
- **Text/Lists**: Text may be simplified with bulleted lists.

### Spreadsheets

Historically, a spreadsheet has been a bookkeeping document—often found in a ledger with two facing pages and columns and cells to enter information. These are still used in some businesses, especially small businesses, but almost all larger businesses utilize an electronic spreadsheet, which is a software application that organizes and stores data (numeric or text) in tables and allows for analysis. Cells in a spreadsheet are arranged in columns and rows. A commonly used spreadsheet is Microsoft Excel. Spreadsheets were originally used primarily for budgetary reasons to track income and expenditures, but use has expanded. For example, spreadsheets are used extensively in education to keep track of assignments and grades and to report grades. They are used in research to keep track of results. If the spreadsheet program is part of a software productivity suite (such as Microsoft Office), then information from the spreadsheet can be easily exported into other applications, such as the word processing program.

### Presentation Software

Presentation software, such as PowerPoint, is often used to supplement lectures or to provide standalone modules. Text is more tiring for the eyes on screen than on the printed page because of the illumination of the screen, and some fonts may blur in browsers, so fonts especially designed for the web, such as Verdana and Lucida Sans/Grande, should be used for text that will be accessed on a browser. Using a variety of fonts and multiple sizes on one screen can be very distracting. Font size should be 12-14 for standard text with greater size for headings. When projected, font size must be large enough to be read easily from the back of the room. Long paragraphs should be avoided and information broken into small chunks with adequate white space to rest the eyes. Text against a colored background, especially a deep color, is difficult to read. When highlighting text, underlining is more evident than italicizing and bolding because screens and projectors have different lighting and resolution. Colored fonts may be used sparingly to highlight different types of information. For example, a question or heading may be in blue and explanations in black fonts.

#### *TEMPLATES*

A template is a file that contains the basic structure of a specific type of document. For example, templates are available in word processing programs for business letters, fax cover sheets, and event calendars. Additionally, numerous templates are available for free online. Templates are available not only for documents but also for websites. People can design templates to meet specific needs, setting up the format, margins, font style, and font size. Once the template is set up, then no further formatting is required. Templates save time and simplify documentation. Templates are especially valuable if different individuals must produce the same type of document because the templates ensure that the individuals will use the same format. Templates make it easier to obtain needed information from a document and to combine information from various documents.

## Technology Tools and Strategies

### LEARNING TECHNOLOGY PRINCIPLES

Learning technology principles include:

- Technology should add value that is evidence-based to the educational process or the activity. Technology should be selected only if it is appropriate for needs and the impact understood.
- The technology utilized should be designed for teaching and learning. Software applications should be designed specifically for education rather than adapted from other uses.
- Standards of quality for the use of technology should be outlined, applied, and monitored.
- Technology should be cost-effective and sustainable with consideration given to the needs of training and upgrades.
- Access to technology should be open to as many as possible.
- Technology should be scalable so new technology can be connected to the existing network, and software should be compatible with other software in use.
- Technology should be utilized in partnership and collaboration to increase access.
- Technology should provide various strategies to appeal to different learning styles.
- Technology should promote lifelong learning.
- Technology should be customizable to meet the needs of different populations and different purposes.

### MULTIMEDIA TECHNOLOGIES

#### *AUDIENCE RESPONSE TOOLS AND SMART BOARDS*

Audience response tools allow for interaction between the presenter and the audience. A typical tool is a small wireless keyboard that the audience member can use to respond, such as by selecting the answer to a multiple-choice question. These devices are often referred to as clickers. A similar virtual audience response tool may be used for online presentations.

SMART boards are interactive white boards that are part of a system that includes a computer and projector. The contents on a computer can be displayed on the SMART board, which is touch sensitive so that the user can write or draw on the image on the board as well. Information is shared between the computer and the SMART board. SMART boards are available in different sizes and with different degrees of interactivity and utilize digital vision touch software to allow response to touch and digital ink.

### *Projectors*

Projectors connect to computers and provide a large display of the content on the computer on a screen. The size of the projected content can often be adjusted for the needs and size of the audience. When choosing a projector, the important information needed is the size of the screen (width) onto which the image will be projected because some projectors may lose focus if the image is too large, the distance from the projector to the screen because this will also affect the clarity of the image, and the amount of light in the room because some projectors must be used in a dark room, especially older projectors. It is important to consider the brightness and resolution as projectors vary widely. Pocket projectors are small and easily transportable but suitable only for small groups and lack brightness and zoom lenses. Multimedia projectors are most commonly used for presentation software but vary in brightness.

## Teaching Strategies Using Technology

### *Virtual Reality*

Virtual reality is a form of learning/gaming in which the individual receives sensory inputs (sounds, visuals) through the computer while sometimes wearing special glasses, earphones, and sometimes special gloves or bodysuits. This immersive technology allows the user to enter a virtual world and practice various skills. Users create avatars to use during participation. Some universities have set up virtual environments in *Second Life*, an online virtual world. Virtual reality has been used to teach learners to carry out procedures, which they can practice in the virtual environment. Virtual reality has been used more commonly with medical students but has many uses for nursing education. Students can participate in virtual simulations and learn from their mistakes without injury to real patients. With virtual reality, the learner can engage in activities that would be too expensive in real life. Another use of virtual reality is for virtual meetings where avatars interact and communicate.

### *Stimulations*

Simulations use real or realistic equipment and materials as part of teaching strategies. As enrollment has increased in nursing programs and nursing care has become more complex, the need for education and practice has expanded, but opportunities for specific types of learning and training are not always readily available, especially with expensive equipment. Technology-based simulations can compensate for that deficit and are especially attractive to the younger generations of learners who have grown up with technology. However, some simulation equipment is also very expensive and requires training, which usually comes at a cost, to program and monitor. Instructors must have good mastery of computer skills, and this can pose problems for some. Simulations can be used with almost all types of medical and nursing education and can be useful adjuncts to clinical experience. Simulations are especially valuable to prepare students for emergency and critical care situations.

### Computer-Assisted Instruction

Computer-assisted instruction (CAI) or computer-based training (CBT) can be used to provide or support course/training content. Advantages to CAI/CBT are that the training is self-paced, allowing the individual flexibility in the speed of learning as well as access, which may be 24 hours daily, especially if internet based. Training can be offered by online and offline. CAI/CBT improves retention, especially when it involves interactivity and is used to teach about technology and facilities mastery by allowing students to review and progress as they are able. To promote effectiveness, learning aids, such as questions and guides, should be prepared in advance and a trainer should be available onsite or online to provide assistance. Some disadvantages include the time involved in preparing CAI/CBT modules and supporting materials and the need to conform to the restrictions of the programmed options.

## Social Networking Tools

### Blogs

Blogs (web logs) are online journals that can be set up for free and to which people can comment. Many are personal blogs, but health-related and support group blogs are increasingly available. However, many of the current health-related blogs are set up by consumers rather than healthcare professionals, so information is not always reliable. While blogs are essentially electronic diaries, they can be easily adapted for educational purposes. Blogs can be set up for all types of learners and for stand-alone content or content in support of other classwork. Blogs can contain text, audio, images, and video, and can link to other websites and blogs.

### Gaming

Gaming is the use of competitive activities to facilitate learning. Gaming may be as simple as word games or very complex computer-based games requiring advanced critical thinking skills. Gaming may be utilized anywhere in teaching, but it is most often used to reinforce learning rather than to introduce new concepts. Edutainment (software applications of education games) is becoming more common and is especially attractive to younger generations who have grown up playing computer games. Gaming may be used for needs and outcomes assessment as well as for instructional purposes. When selecting edutainment software, the instructor should evaluate the suitability of the software application to determine if it meets objectives, the games can be completed in an allotted time period, and the layout is conducive to learning. The instructor should consider how many can play the game at one time and issues of access as well as costs.

### Social Network Sites

Social network sites are usually modern sites. The primary characteristic of a modern site is interactivity. Instead of the application being on the individual's computer, it is based on the internet. Typical modern sites include social media (such as Facebook) that allow users to manipulate data and comment as well as YouTube, which allows users to watch and upload videos. Commonly used social network sites include:

- LinkedIn is a network designed for professionals and professional communications. Members are able to access information about jobs, current trends, and professional news, as well as information about marketing.
- Facebook is an open social media site that is used for personal communications as well as special-interest groups but is less focused on business.
- Twitter allows instant messages to followers. While originally limited to 140 characters, this limitation has been relaxed.

When initiating a social media site to provide information about a healthcare organization and to allow feedback, the best way of handling feedback from the public is to monitor and censor if inappropriate.

## Clinical Technologies

### *Smart Pumps and Point-of-Care Scanners*

Smart pumps include infusion pumps for large volumes and syringes as well as for patient-controlled analgesia. Smart pumps are programmable and sound alarms if problems, such as completion of an IV, arise. Smart pumps are increasingly sophisticated and some can interact with the patient's electronic health record as well as the CPOE and barcode medication scanner. Some have built-in drug libraries (error reduction software) to monitor dosage and frequency of drugs. Smart pumps reduce errors, but they can be programmed incorrectly and alarms ignored or overridden, so they are not error proof.

Scanners include large CT scanner and MRI scanner as well as ultrasound equipment, but smaller scanners are available for clinical application. These include bladder scanners, which allow the nurse to scan the patient's bladder at the point of care to determine if the bladder is full or distended and to determine post-voiding retention.

### *Barcode Medication Scanners*

Barcode medication administration (BCMA) utilizes wireless mobile units at the point of care to scan the barcode on each unit of medication or blood component before it is dispensed. Scanning ensures the correct medication and dosage is given to the correct patient, eliminating most point of administration medication errors. The BCMA system can also be utilized for specimen collection. This system requires monitoring and input from the pharmacy, as each new barcode must be entered into the system. Additionally, some medications are received in bulk, so when they are dispensed in unit doses, barcodes must be individually attached. Staff must be trained to ensure that BCMA is utilized properly and consistently. The FDA has required that drug supplies provide barcodes on the labels of medications and other biological product. BCMA increases safety for patients, and integrates with the medication administration record and the information system of the organization, providing data for assessment of performance and performance improvement measures.

### *Radiofrequency Identification*

Radiofrequency identification (RFI) is an automatic system for identification that employs embedded digital memory chips, with unique codes, to track patients, medical devices, medications, and staff. A chip can carry multiple types of data, such as expiration dates, patient's allergies, and blood types. A chip/tag may, for example, be embedded in the identification bracelet of the patient and all medications for the patient tagged with the same chip. Chips have the ability to both read and write data, so they are more flexible than bar coding. The data on the chips can be read by sensors from a distance or through materials, such as clothes, although tags do not apply or read well on metal or in fluids. There are two types of RFI:

- **Active**: Continuous signals are transmitted between the chips and sensors.
- **Passive**: Signals are transmitted when in close proximity to a sensor.

Thus, a passive system may be adequate for administration of medications, but an active system would be needed to track movements of staff, equipment, or patients.

### *Handheld Devices*

Handheld devices include smartphones, mobile phones, tablets (such as the iPad), netbooks, iPod, iPod Touch, personal digital assistants (PDAs), Nintendo DS, and educational personal assistants (EPAs). These devices are easily accessible, portable, and in common use. One advantage is that they can be accessed at any time. In some cases, educational content is available for specific devices (such as the smartphone and iPad). Handheld devices can be used to access content on the internet and to download prepared materials (websites, articles, videos, pictures, ebooks) and allow for viewing videos and listening to podcasts. The devices allow interactivity to varying degrees and allow the learner to email or respond to others. They may allow direct access to patient records. Many companies now offer software and a wide range of educational materials specifically for handheld technologies, supporting various learning styles and allowing for tracking of learner participation. Handheld devices can also be used to document patient care and access clinical data.

# Program/Project Management and Process Improvement

## Performance Improvement Methodologies

### PDCA/PDSA

Plan-Do-Check (Study)-Act (PDCA/PDSA) (Shewhart cycle) is a method of continuous quality improvement. PDCA is simple and understandable; however, it may be difficult to maintain this cycle consistently because of lack of focus and commitment. PDCA may be more suited to solving specific problems than organization-wide problems:

- **Plan**: Identifying, analyzing, and defining the problem, setting goals, and establishing a process that coordinates with leadership. Extensive brainstorming, including fishbone diagrams, identifies problematic processes and lists current process steps. Data are collected and analyzed and root cause analysis completed.
- **Do**: Generating solutions from which to select one or more and then implementing the solution on a trial basis.
- **Check**: Gathering and analyzing data to determine the effectiveness of the solution. If effective, then continue to *Act*; if not, return to *Plan* and pick a different solution. (*Study* may replace *Check: PDSA.)*
- **Act**: Identifying changes that need to be done to fully implement solution, adopting solution, and continuing to monitor results while picking another improvement project.

### Six Sigma

Six Sigma is a performance improvement model developed by Motorola to improve business practices and increase profits. This model has been adapted to many types of businesses, including health care. Six Sigma is a data-driven performance model that aims to eliminate "defects" in processes that involve products or services. The goal is to achieve Six Sigma, meaning no more than 3.4 defects per 1 million opportunities. This program focuses on continuous improvement with the customer's perception as key, so that the customer defines that which is "critical to quality" (CTQ). Two different types of improvement projects may be employed: DMAIC (define, measure, analyze, improve, control) for existing processes or products that need improvement and DMADV (define, measure, analyze, design, verify) for development of new high-quality processes or products. Both DMAIC and DMADV utilize trained personnel to execute the plans. These personnel use martial arts titles: green belts, black belts (execute programs), and master black belts (supervise programs).

### Six Sigma DMAIC

The first model for **Six Sigma** is DMAIC (define, measure, analyze, improve, control), and it is used when existing processes or products need improvement and in healthcare quality:

- **Define** costs and benefits that will be achieved when changes instituted. Develop list of customer needs based on complaints, requests.
- **Measure** input, process, and output measure, collect baseline date, establish costs, and perform analysis, calculate sigma rating.
- **Analyze** root or other causes of current defects, use data to confirm, and uncover steps in processes that are counterproductive.

- **Improve** by creating potential solutions, develop and pilot plans, implement, and measure results, determining cost savings and other benefits to customers.
- **Control** includes standardizing work processes and monitoring the system by linking performance measures to a balanced scorecard, creating processes for updating procedures, disseminating reports, and recommending future processes.

### Lean Six Sigma

Lean Six Sigma, a method that combines Six Sigma with concepts of "lean" thinking, is a method of focusing process improvement on strategic goals rather than on a project-by-project basis. This type of program is driven by strong senior leadership that outlines long-term goals and strategies. Physicians are an important part of the process and must be included and engaged. The basis of this program is to reduce error and waste within the organization through continuous learning and rapid change. There are four characteristics:

- Long-term goals with strategies in place for 1- to 3-year periods.
- Performance improvement is the underlying belief system.
- Cost reduction through quality increase, supported by statistics evaluating the cost of inefficiency.
- Incorporation of improvement methodology, such as DMAIC, PDCA, or other methods.

### Role of Champions and Team Leaders in Performance Improvement Measures

Champions are those individuals with a particular passion for or interest in the activities of a performance improvement team and are often instrumental in the creation and formation of the teams themselves, choosing the basic function of the team and the team members. Because members of organizations are often very resistive to change, the champion has a pivotal role in providing leadership. This process champion (also called a sponsor) is often a member of upper management with the authority to make decisions and the ability to communicate with top management and the governing board. Champions may exist at different levels as well, so there may be clinical champions or patient safety champions, individuals who have made an effort to be informed and to promote performance improvement.

The process owners, on the other hand, are usually the team leaders, who are actively involved in supervising and/or carrying out the functions and activities of the team. Process owners are often key managers with knowledge and commitment to improvement.

## Indicators, Priorities, and Trends

### Joint Commission's Core Measures

The Joint Commission has established **National Quality Core Measures** to determine if healthcare institutions are in compliance with current standards based on CMS quality indicators. The Core Measures involve a series of questions that are answered either "yes" or "no" to indicate if an action was completed. There are now 15 Core Measure sets:

- Cardiac Care
- Assisted living community measures
- Health care staffing services
- Hospital-based inpatient psychiatric services (HBIPS)
- Hospital outpatient department measures
- Palliative care

- Perinatal care
- Stroke
- Spine Surgery
- Venous thromboembolism (VTE)
- Emergency department
- Immunization
- Substance use
- Tobacco treatment
- Total hip and knee replacement

For each condition, questions relate to whether or not standard care was provided, such as whether a stroke patient was discharged on antithrombic therapy. The data are public and provide useful information about these particular standards, but do not necessarily reflect the overall quality of care, so these measurements alone are not adequate performance measures but must be considered along with other indicators.

## Retention and Nursing Satisfaction

Nursing has been plagued with a shortage of personnel, which poses a risk to patient care, and high rates of turnover with attendant costs in orienting and training new staff. **Retention** is, therefore, a critical concern. Retention estimates can be made through assessing potential retirements and conducting a **nursing satisfaction** survey to identify problem areas. Key elements to staff retention include:

- Providing competitive salaries and benefits
- Establishing a thorough orientation program, including mentoring
- Developing support and preceptoring programs for new graduate nurses
- Providing flexible work schedules
- Offering health and wellness programs
- Ensuring adequate staffing
- Providing staff training and career development programs
- Hiring recently retired staff consultant or part-time work
- Offering educational incentives, such as tuition assistance, to promote advancement and certification
- Encouraging collaboration and team building as well as nursing autonomy and decision making
- Recognizing professional excellence

## Patient Satisfaction

Patient/customer satisfaction is usually measured with surveys given to patients upon discharge from an institution or on completion of treatment. One problem with analyzing surveys is that establishing benchmarks can be difficult because so many different survey and data collection methods are used that comparison data may be meaningless. Internal benchmarking may be more effective, but the sample rate for surveys may not be sufficient to provide validity. As patients become more knowledgeable and the demand for accountability increases, patient satisfaction is being used as a guide for performance improvement, although patient perceptions of clinical care do not always correlate with outcomes. The results of surveys can provide feedback that makes healthcare providers more aware of customer expectations. Currently, surveys are most often used to evaluate service elements of care rather than clinical elements. Analysis includes:

- Determining the patient/customer's degree of trust
- Determining the degree of satisfaction with care/treatment
- Identifying needs that may be unmet
- Identifying patient/customer priorities

## Nursing Sensitive Indicators

In 1994, the American Nurses Association (ANA) began to investigate the impact that healthcare restructuring had on patient care, identifying nurse-sensitive indicators. Nurse-sensitive indicators are the elements of care—process, outcomes, and structures—related specifically to nursing. Indicators should be able to be tracked and evaluated and may focus on the following:

- **Patient-focused outcomes**: Measurable outcomes, such as rate of urinary tract infections, pressure ulcers, falls, patient injuries, and patient satisfaction with care (pain control, nursing response, and education). These outcomes should improve with increased quality or quantity of nursing care.
- **Process of care**: Methods used to provide care (such as routine infection control measures) and staff satisfaction. These processes should improve with better education, supervision, mentoring, and feedback.
- **Structure**: Staffing ratios (such as registered nurses [RNs] to licensed vocational nurses [LVNs] to certified nursing assistants [CNAs]), total hours of nursing care per patient per day, nurse turnover, and nursing education and certification. An improvement in structure often requires increased financial and/or time investment and evidence of cost-effectiveness.

## Dashboards

A dashboard (also called a digital dashboard), like the dashboard in a car, is an easy to access and read computer program that integrates a variety of performance measures or key indicators into one display (usually with graphs or charts) to provide an overview of an organization. It might include data regarding patient satisfaction, infection rates, financial status, or any other measurement that is important to assess performance. The dashboard provides a running picture of the status of the department or organization at any point in time, and may be updated as desired: daily, weekly, or monthly. An organization-wide dashboard provides numerous benefits, including the following:

- Broad involvement of all departments
- A consistent and easy-to-understand visual representation of data
- Identification of negative findings or trends so that they can be corrected
- Availability of detailed reports
- Effective measurements that demonstrate the degree of efficiency
- Assistance with making informed decisions

## Balanced Scorecards

The balanced scorecard (designed by Kaplan and Norton) is based on the strategic plan and provides performance measures in relation to the mission and vision statement and goals and objectives. A balanced scorecard includes not only the traditional financial information but also includes data about customers, internal processes, and education/learning. Each organization can select measures that help to determine if the organization is on track to meeting its goals. These measures may include:

- **Customers**: Types of customers and customer satisfaction.
- **Finances/business operations**: Financial data may include funding and cost-benefit analysis.
- **Clinical outcomes**: Complications, infection rates, inpatient and outpatient data, and compliance with regulatory standards.
- **Education/learning**: In-service training, continuing education, assessment of learning and utilization of new skills, and research.
- **Community**: Ongoing needs.
- **Growth**: Innovative programs.

If the scorecard is adequately balanced, it will reflect both the needs and priorities of the organization itself and also those of the community and customers.

## Interpretation and Incorporation of Data

### Incorporating Performance Improvement Data into Professional Development

Incorporating performance improvement data should be central to all work of the nursing professional development specialist and data should be routinely disseminated as part of practice, education, and consultation. Any time the specialist gives a presentation or provides written material, references should be made to research findings because this provides supporting evidence and lends credence to the information the nurse is providing. Often, research can provide guidance for surveillance or interventions and give valuable insights. References that are used or referred to should always be properly cited so that the work of researchers is credited. If a presentation is given orally, then the nurse should prepare a list of references. Newsletters and email or internet reports and communications should include research highlights or summaries of current studies of interest, with links to online articles provided, when possible, to encourage people to read the research for themselves and become more knowledgeable about issues related to patients.

### Interpreting and Incorporating Data to Inform Decision Making

When engaged in decision making, the first step is to ask the right question and then to search for the best possible evidence, beginning with database and journal searches, and to rate the level of evidence, keeping in mind that meta-analysis and randomized controlled trials are strong evidence and expert opinion is weak. It is important to search a number of different sources in order to find information that is relevant, including both internal sources (such as electronic health records) and external sources. Once data are located, then they must be interpreted to determine if the data have external validity and can apply to the question at hand. Data should be carefully reviewed to determine how the research converges or diverges from the current issue. Final decisions should be made in collaboration with others after review of the evidence so that there is consensus.

### Aligning Professional Development with Priorities, Initiative, and Trends

Nursing professional development activities should align with the following:

- **Organizational priorities**: These are often outlined by the board of directors and administration, and are associated with the mission and vision statements of the organization, so these priorities often are more broad than others and developed through discussion and/or mandate.

- **Departmental priorities**: These priorities tend to focus on immediate needs, such as efforts to reduce infections or decrease error, and interests of staff members, and are developed through collaboration.
- **Initiatives**: Initiatives may be local, state, or federal, and are usually communicated through the media and may or may not require specific types of activities.
- **Performance trends**: These may be organizational performance trends, but these trends are most often compared with national trends compiled by government or professional organizations. Often, extensive research is available regarding performance trends to help in developing activities.

# Project Management

## Elements of the Project Plan

Elements of the project plan include plans for and management of the following:

- **Purpose**: What will be achieved by the project.
- **Scope**: General work to be done and/or end product, department involvement/responsibilities.
- **Requirements**: Agreed upon documentation, agreements, tracing, and reporting.
- **Schedule of activities**: Includes activities, milestones, products, and timeline.
- **Finances**: Explanation of budget, financial resources, payroll, potential unexpected expenses.
- **Quality control**: Monitoring, reporting, and correcting for quality issues.
- **Resources**: Materials, staff, equipment, finances needed to complete the project, and expected utilization of resources.
- **Stakeholders**: Identification of stakeholders, prioritizing stakeholders, methods of communication with and management of stakeholders.
- **Risks**: Anticipating and identifying risk factors, methods to manage and respond to risks and reduce liability.
- **Communications**: Plans for internal and external communication, including public relations.
- **Purchasing**: Vendors, cost-comparison, methods of purchase, timeline for purchase, inventory.
- **Change**: Requirements for and response to change in plans.

## Project Management

### *Stakeholders*

Stakeholders are those who are actively involved in a project or in some way affected or impacted by a project. Stakeholders in project management are often numerous and varied and can include sponsors, project managers, members of the project team, support staff, suppliers, customers, users, and even opponents. It is important for the project manager to identify stakeholders and to develop a stakeholder management strategy. Creating a stakeholder registry that lists all stakeholders and includes details about the stakeholders, such as their level of interest or influence, can be helpful but it is often kept confidential. As part of stakeholder management, the project manager should note what type of feedback and frequency of contact is appropriate for each stakeholder. For example, the sponsor may require a weekly update, but the supplier may need to be contacted only prior to needed delivery of supplies.

### SUSTAINABILITY

Project management has three primary **constraints** that must be considered if the project and outcomes are to have sustainability:

- **Scope**: This is essentially the goal of the project, the end product, or services that will be produced, and includes the work to be done and the methods that will be used to verify the scope.
- **Timeline**: This includes the schedule of activities and expected duration of the project. The methods used to track actual schedule performance should be outlined as well as the approval required to alter or change the timeline.
- **Finances**: This includes the source of funding and the actual budget for the project. The method for tracking the budget and expenses should be clearly outlined as well as any reporting requirements. Information should include who can authorize changes to the budget and what procedures must be followed.

### DEVELOPING A TIMELINE

The purpose of developing a timeline as part of project management is to ensure that the project is completed in a timely manner and that activities are coordinated. Initial processes involved include the following:

- Identify and define activities or tasks that must be performed and create an activities list that describes attributes of the activity.
- Create a milestone list based on the activities.
- Sequence the activities, showing the relationship between different activities, and create project schedule diagrams.
- Estimate activity resources (staff, equipment, materials) needed to perform activities by creating a document outlining resource needs.
- Estimate duration of activities by estimating and documenting the time needed for each activity.
- Develop the schedule: Use a method, such as Gantt chart, to create the project schedule and show the sequence of activities, including those that are concurrent or overlapping.
- Control the schedule: Manage changes, resources, change requests, and resource utilization.

#### GANTT CHART

A Gantt chart is used for developing improvement projects to manage schedules and estimate time needed to complete tasks. It is a bar chart with a horizontal time scale that presents a visual representation of the beginning and end points of time when different steps in a process should be completed. Gantt charts are a component of project management software programs. The Gantt chart is usually created after initial brainstorming, and creation of a timeline and action plans. Steps to creation of a Gantt chart include:

1. List the name of the process at the top.
2. Create a chart with a timeline of days, weeks, months (as appropriate for process) horizontally across the top.
3. List tasks vertically on the left of the chart.

4. Draw horizontal lines/bars with from the expected beginning point to the expected end point for each task. These may be color-coded to indicate which individual/team is responsible for completing the task.

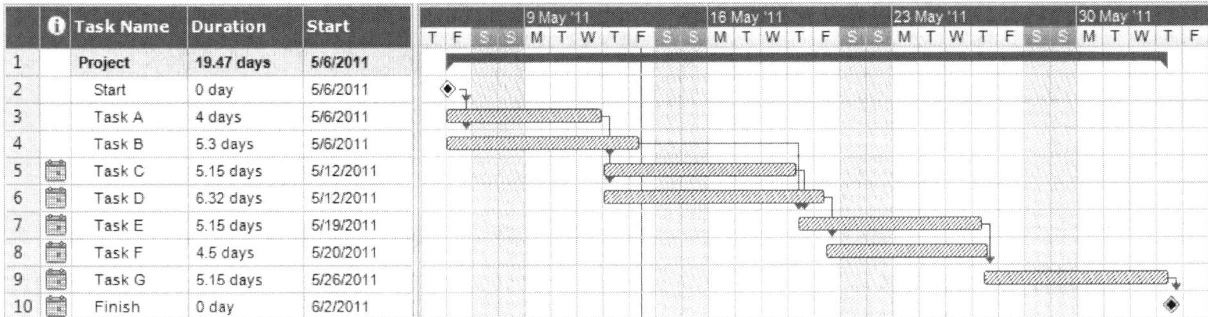

| | | Task Name | Duration | Start |
|---|---|---|---|---|
| 1 | | Project | 19.47 days | 5/6/2011 |
| 2 | | Start | 0 day | 5/6/2011 |
| 3 | | Task A | 4 days | 5/6/2011 |
| 4 | | Task B | 5.3 days | 5/6/2011 |
| 5 | | Task C | 5.15 days | 5/12/2011 |
| 6 | | Task D | 6.32 days | 5/12/2011 |
| 7 | | Task E | 5.15 days | 5/19/2011 |
| 8 | | Task F | 4.5 days | 5/20/2011 |
| 9 | | Task G | 5.15 days | 5/26/2011 |
| 10 | | Finish | 0 day | 6/2/2011 |



## CRITICAL PATH METHOD, CRITICAL CHAIN, AND PERT TECHNIQUE

**Critical path method** is a network diagramming technique used to estimate the total duration of a project. The project manager develops a diagram that shows all of the primary paths with estimated duration of time for each and then identifies the longest path through the network design. This, in turn, provides the earliest time by which the project can be completed. Slack or float refers to amount of delay time that an activity can be delayed without impacting the overall completion time.

**Critical chain scheduling** involves identifying constraints and scheduling accordingly. Critical chain scheduling builds in a time buffer for project completion and discourages multitasking, favoring completion of one task before beginning another.

**Program Evaluation and Review Technique (PERT)** is a technique utilized for project time management. PERT is used to estimate times when the duration of individual activities is uncertain. PERT achieves probabilistic time estimates by taking into consideration optimistic, most likely, and pessimistic time estimates.

### *DEVELOPING ACTION PLANS*

Development of performance improvement actions plans usually begins with prioritizing problems after an initial period of monitoring and assessment. Steps include:

1. Utilize systematic approaches to identifying reasons for variation in process, conduct a root cause analysis, and identify feasible changes in process.
2. Formulate an action plan the clearly outlines the expected outcomes, steps in the plan, responsibility, timeline, and types of measurements to use for monitoring and evaluating.
3. Conduct pilot testing after determining time frame, size of sample, and locations.
4. Analyze data from pilot testing.
5. Modify the action plan if indicated and conduct further pilot testing.
6. Commit to action plan: individuals, departments, and areas involved in the process as well as the appropriate leadership/council.
7. Begin to implement the action plan on a limited trial basis after considering and providing for training, education, and scheduling.
8. Determine the most effective performance measures.
9. Establish a timeline for full implementation.
10. Evaluate the trial implementation and make changes or do further analysis as indicated.

### *Measuring and Monitoring*

Measuring and monitoring of a project are ongoing procedures that evaluate progress toward objectives and indicate any deviations so that corrections can be made. Processes vary according to the knowledge area of the project. For example, costs should be compared with the forecast budget and any change requests to determine if there are cost overruns. Activities on the timeline should be assessed to determine if they are on schedule, ahead of schedule, or behind schedule. Risks should be assessed and managed. Changes should be assessed through integrated change control and all change requests documented as well as their approval or rejection. Quality control measurements should be carried out and any defects noted and corrected. Performance of team members should be monitored. Any changes in the scope of a project should be noted and the project plan updated. Performance reports should be completed as scheduled and disseminated to the proper individuals or agencies.

### *Funding Opportunities*

Funding is always a major concern of project management. Funding opportunities include:

- **Home organization**: An appeal to the board of directors, outlining the purpose and benefits of a program may convince the board to fund a project.
- **Community agencies/organizations**: If a project meets community needs, agencies or organizations in the community may be willing to provide partial or complete funding and may be willing to partner with the project manager.
- **Government grants**: Local, state, and national government programs often provide grants for healthcare projects. In some cases, the grants are for specific types of projects; in other cases, the project manager may submit a proposal. AHRQ maintains the Grants online Database (GOLD) where the project manager can search for grant and funding opportunities.
- **Private**: Private individuals or companies may be willing to fund projects as an act of philanthropy or, in some cases, as an act of self-interest, depending on what they expect in return

### *Customer Service*

Customer service is an important part of the project manager's duties. The project manager should identify exactly who the customer is at the onset of a project and determine the customer needs. The first step in customer service is to listen actively to the customer, asking questions if necessary and showing concern. The project manager should communicate clearly in terms the customer can understand and provide written documentation when indicated. The project manager should maintain up-to-date records of any customer complaints, requests, or concerns to save time on follow-up contacts and to help validate the customer's concerns. Resolutions should also be recorded. One of the most important aspects of customer service is to attend to customers' needs in a timely manner because delays often lead to increased conflict and problems.

### ELEMENTS OF THE BUSINESS PLAN

Elements of the business plan include the following:

| | |
|---|---|
| **Executive summary** | Outline all of the key elements to the business proposal, including the customer, product/services, goals, risks, opportunities, costs, management, and timeline. |
| **Product/Service** | Provide a detailed description but avoid being overly technical, including the ways in which this product/service compares with others. Note the need for patents, licenses, or any regulatory requirements. |
| **Management** | Explain the hierarchy and division of duties, including explanation of professional experience and education. |
| **Market Survey** | Discuss similar products/services, target groups, and projected market volume. |
| **Marketing strategies** | Explain placement, promotion, and pricing. |
| **Organization** | Describe structure of business, provide flow charts, and describe production capability, costs, quality assurance methods, and inventory (if appropriate). |
| **Timeline** | Describe the timeline for implementation from beginning to fully operational business. |
| **Risk factors** | Describe both opportunities from gain and risk factors that may impact product/sales and methods to deal with risk factors. |
| **Appendices** | Provide samples of forms and any additional information that is necessary. |

## Program Management

### PROMOTIONAL STRATEGIES

#### *MARKETING STRATEGIES*

The first task in the development of a marketing strategy is to determine the objectives and the target market. Market research may involve literature review, surveys, questionnaires, market analysis, and focus groups. The target market may be segmented according to various demographics with each segment requiring a different approach. The marketing plan should include different marketing strategies: advertisements (print, TV, radio), direct marketing, trade shows/conferences. SWOT analysis is often done to determine the strengths and weaknesses of an organization as part of the marketing plan. If a product is involved, then product research must be conducted. Benchmarking through tracking such as by using web analytics to determine traffic on a website or by list splitting (different versions of a mailer sent to different populations), can help to provide useful data. In some cases, the best initial marketing strategy may be to utilize a market research agency to gather information.

#### SWOT ANALYSIS

SWOT analysis is commonly used to help determine an organization's strengths and weaknesses and as part of strategic planning; however, SWOT analysis can be used for any type of decision making as it provides a good overview of the organization and helps to provide an outline of different factors affecting decisions. SWOT analysis is often done as part of market planning as preparation for carrying out a marketing program. SWOT analysis considers the strengths and weaknesses of the internal environment and the opportunities and threats of the external environment:

| Internal environment | | External environment | |
|---|---|---|---|
| **Strengths** | **Weaknesses** | **Opportunities** | **Threats** |
| Financial stability<br>Programs and services<br>Staff persons<br>Client/Staff satisfaction | Increasing costs<br>Outdated equipment<br>Ineffective programs<br>Marketing | Increased population<br>New programs<br>New markets<br>Stakeholders | Low reimbursement<br>Regulations<br>Competition<br>Political changes |

### *Public Relations*

Public relations is the process involved in maintaining a good public image through the management of information about and between the organization and the public or other organizations. While public relations shares some aspects with marketing, public relations is not intended to directly sell a product but to maintain good relations, which may in turn enhance marketing strategies. The initial step in public relations is to identify the public, which, in fact, may be multiple (individuals, organizations, government agencies, accreditation agencies, vendors). Different public entities require targeted messages. Media coverage is often part of public relations and the primary means of communicating achievements, but information released to general media (such as TV, newspapers, and radio) should be geared toward the reader/viewer and is usually less detailed than that for professional media (journals). Strong visuals should be used whenever possible. As part of public relations, the organization should also target special events, such as health fairs and public health initiatives.

## Program Evaluation

### *Measurement*

The purpose of program evaluation is to determine if the program is working effectively by assessing whether objectives are being met. As part of program evaluation, performance measures are carried out to evaluate measurable outcomes. Different approaches to program evaluation include:

- **Process**: The purpose is to determine if the program is operating as planned and generally looks at activities and whether the program meets regulatory requirements and professional standards.
- **Outcome**: The purpose is to determine the effectiveness of the program by assessing whether the outputs and outcomes of a program are as intended or if there are unexpected results.
- **Impact**: The purpose is to attempt to determine the effectiveness of the program by assessing the difference between the outcomes and what would likely have occurred without the program.
- **Cost-benefit/Cost-effectiveness**: Cost-benefit analysis looks at all costs and benefits associated with the program to determine whether or not there is benefit. Cost-effectiveness analysis, on the other hand, looks at the cost effectiveness of individual aspects of the program.

### *Principles of Monitoring*

Monitoring is an essential part of program evaluation and should be an ongoing process throughout the life of a program. Monitoring principles include:

- Monitoring should compare current status with baseline data. Baseline data should be used to set targets for improvement.
- Monitoring should determine whether or not progress is being made.
- Monitoring should be planned as an integral part of every program.
- Monitoring and evaluating should be planned together at the same time.
- Information derived from monitoring should be utilized in making decisions.
- The methodology for monitoring should be clearly outlined and followed consistently.
- Monitoring should be carried out in a manner that protects confidentiality.
- Monitoring should assess all primary stakeholders.
- Monitoring should be scheduled on a routine basis.
- A monitoring matrix should be developed to facilitate monitoring.
- Resources for monitoring should be separate from other program resources.

## Management of Resources

### *Personnel, Finances, and Data*

Resource management requires effective use of resources when and where they are needed in an organization or institution. Resource management in health care should include a focus on both current and future (or emergency) needs.

| Resource | Issues |
|---|---|
| **Personnel** | **Staffing levels**: Numbers, licensed vs unlicensed, administrative vs. support, permanent vs part-time<br>**Assignments**: Permanent vs floating, allocation, flexibility<br>**Training**: Ongoing, continuing education, orientation<br>**Supervision**: Hierarchy, evaluation procedures, disciplinary procedures<br>**Regulations**: Compliance, education, ADA |
| **Finances** | **Resource leveling**: Balancing supply and demand with maintenance of inventories<br>**Accounting practices**: Types of budgets<br>**Costs vs revenue**: Direct and indirect costs, grants, claims and payments, net vs. gross<br>**Regulations**: Reporting requirements, tax implications |
| **Data** | **Data collection**: Responsibility, methods, frequency, duration, database design, local vs system<br>**Analysis**: Methods, benchmarking, cost-effectiveness<br>**Utilization**: Process improvement, allocation of resources<br>**Dissemination**: Extent, method<br>**Regulations**: HIPAA, state and federal |

### *Resource Utilization*

Resource utilization refers to the consideration of all factors related to the planning and delivery of quality professional development activities. Resources may be allotted to the physical environment for building or remodeling, staffing, equipment, literature, training, and outreach programs. Utilization review requires consideration of individual safety, program effectiveness, and cost.

Interventions should be safe, effective, and affordable for each individual. Decisions should take into consideration rising healthcare costs and how to maximize the use of resources while continuing to provide quality professional development activities. The goal of resource utilization is to provide quality, cost-effective programs while using the best-qualified staff and appropriate resources.

### *Facility Management*

Facility management requires not only attention to operational issues, such as compliance with state or federal regulations regarding safety issues and budget management, but also strategic issues, such as utilization of space and services. Supporting business operations and ensuring adequate maintenance of the facility are paramount. Issues include:

- **Health and safety**: Compliance with OSHA and EPA requirements, control of hazardous substances/materials, air quality, heating and air conditioning, and safety rules.
- **Fire prevention/safety**: Smoke detectors, fire extinguishers, sprinkler systems, fire doors, evacuation plans, and alarms.
- **Safety/security**: Locks, alarms, security officers, and closed-circuit TV monitoring systems.
- **Inspections**: Regular maintenance and inspection of equipment and environment, including facility and outside spaces.
- **Operations**: Waste management, janitorial services, pest control, access, utilities, scheduling, meeting vendors, ordering, lease of space, and budget management.

### *Staffing*

Staffing management involves both clinical staff (such as nurses) and nonclinical staff (such as housekeeping staff and office personnel). Issues include:

- Workforce size and distribution, including full-time equivalent staff members (one or a combination of more than one staff member who works 80 hours in 14 days) required.
- Educational resources (training programs) and availability of trained personnel (including professional staff and support staff).
- Staff training and ongoing need for staff development and opportunities for certification or advancement.
- Demographics: Population (age, economic levels, ethnic backgrounds, lifestyles) affects the need for care.
- Incentives for career advancement, including increases in income, promotion, and certification.
- Staff turnover/burnout and ongoing need for recruitment.
- Organizational structure.
- Financial resources available.
- Cost-effective staffing, billable provision of care.
- Reimbursement (Medicare, Medicaid, health insurance, or private pay).
- Supervision/feedback.
- Strategies for staffing (organization-wide).

### Scheduling and Other Activities

Once the schedule and timeline are completed, the project manager must control the schedule and activities involved. The primary goal is to be aware of the schedule status and minimize but manage changes. Some tools and techniques used in schedule control include:

- Requiring regular progress reports
- Utilizing a schedule change control system
- Monitoring schedule comparison bar charts (such as Gantt)
- Analyzing slack, leads, and lags
- Carrying out performance measures
- Utilizing resource leveling

The project manager must assess the schedule to determine if the timeline is realistic because it if is not, the project will be delayed, and this can result in problems with administration. The project manager must keep administration apprised of the status of the schedule and the project. The project manager should establish firm dates for key project milestones, as this tends to keep others on track.

### Event Management

Event management requires careful planning and control of resources. Steps include:

1. Clearly identify the event and the goals of the event as well as any constraints (budget, time, venue). Team members should be selected and all tasks identified and assigned.
2. Establish a schedule that sets deadlines and specific milestone (such as the date a speaker must be paid or catering must be contracted for).
3. Communicate with all necessary stakeholders. This includes initial communication with team members and contract individuals, clarifying roles. Communication requirements change as the event is planned and presented.
4. Keep team members involved and delegate tasks as appropriate.
5. Monitor progress. A project management tool, such as Trello or Asana, may be helpful. Gantt charts help to provide a visual image of progress.
6. Maintain flexibility but exhibit leadership and maintain control of preparations for the event.
7. Monitor the event.
8. Debrief to discuss the event and both successful and unsuccessful aspects.

# Nursing Professional Development Practice Test

Want to take this practice test in an online interactive format?
Check out the bonus page, which includes interactive practice questions and much more: **https://www.mometrix.com/bonus948/nursingprofdev**

**1. During what phase of the traditional project life cycle does the project manager provide an accurate estimate of cost and performance reports to stakeholders?**

a. Concept
b. Development
c. Implementation
d. Close-out

**2. If a new type of electronic device is available for healthcare networks, the most important initial consideration for its purchase is:**

a. the life expectancy of the device
b. device integration
c. cost-effectiveness
d. ease of use

**3. If the nursing professional development (NPD) practitioner is applying for a grant through the Health Resources and Services Administration (HRSA) or other government agencies, approximately how much time should be allotted to complete the grant application?**

a. 10 hours
b. 20 hours
c. 40 hours
d. 100 hours

**4. According to Afaf Meleis's transitions theory regarding change, transition conditions include:**

a. facilitators and inhibitors
b. process indicators and outcome indicators
c. critical points or marker events
d. awareness and engagement

**5. Which site provides a hospital report card that shows achievement toward standards in multiple areas including specific surgical procedures, such as total hip replacement and pancreatic resection for cancer?**

a. Centers for Medicare & Medicaid Services (CMS) Care Compare
b. Leapfrog Hospital Safety Grade rankings
c. National Committee for Quality Assurance report cards
d. Healthgrades

**6. The five rights of delegation include the right task, circumstance, person, direction, and:**

a. authority
b. responsibility
c. time frame
d. supervision

**7. When conducting a review of literature as part of the research of best practices, the first thing to consider is the:**

a. source of the material
b. author's credentials
c. thesis
d. evidence

**8. If using critical chain scheduling to ensure that a project with limited resources is completed on time, at the end of the project, it is necessary to include a:**

a. feedback buffer
b. task buffer
c. project buffer
d. resource buffer

**9. The type of conflict most often addressed in conflict-of-interest policies is:**

a. personal
b. financial
c. familial
d. duty

**10. The most effective way to monitor performance is through:**

a. observation
b. personal interviews
c. self-assessments
d. data collection

**11. The first step in succession planning is to:**

a. describe the behaviors, skills, and leadership qualities needed for the role
b. develop a formal written succession plan
c. develop plans for emergency and planned succession
d. outline the needs of the organization

**12. According to the NPD Scope and Standards of Practice, for standard 1, "Assessment of practice gaps," one of the roles of the NPD practitioner is to:**

a. identify the desired outcomes
b. integrate ethics into practice
c. analyze trends and supporting data
d. maintain current knowledge

**13. The primary focus in coaching should be on:**

a. pointing out areas of weakness or errors
b. watching the learner carry out demonstrations
c. developing goals for the learner
d. using questioning to help learners recognize problem areas

**14. Which of the following is a critical element of virtual learning?**

a. Interactivity
b. Scheduled break times
c. Detailed outline
d. Vocabulary list

**15. When developing a promotional strategy, the first step is to determine the:**

a. target audience
b. organizational goals
c. marketing channels
d. costs of different approaches

**16. CMS requires that medical records pertaining to billed services for Medicare Parts A and B be maintained for:**

a. 2 years from the date of service
b. 5 years from the date of service
c. 7 years from the date of service
d. 10 years from the date of service

**17. Which type of database arranges data in rows and columns?**

a. Hierarchical
b. Columnar
c. NoSQL
d. Relational

**18. If the NPD practitioner presents a potential decision but seeks input from staff or teams before making the final decision based on this input, the leadership style is characterized as:**

a. democratic
b. participatory
c. consultative
d. bureaucratic

**19. If a hospital experiences a data breach involving 120 patients and was only able to reach 100 patients by mail or email to notify them, what further action must the hospital take?**

a. Telephone the remaining 20 patients.
b. No further action is required.
c. Post a notice with a toll-free number on the organization's website.
d. Notify the Department of Health and Human Services that 20 patients are unreachable.

**20. According to Albert Bandura's theory of social learning, learning develops from observation, organizing, and rehearsing behavior that has been:**

a. modeled
b. inferred
c. rewarded
d. socially accepted

**21. Risk management's primary responsibility toward incident reports is to:**

a. initiate the incident report
b. assign blame for the incident
c. determine the financial costs of the incident
d. review incident reports to identify possible failures in the system

**22. The primary purpose of multifactor authentication is to:**

a. simplify data protection
b. prevent data breaches
c. encrypt data
d. facilitate data sharing

**23. The NPD practitioner plans to convene a focus group and knows that focus groups usually comprise:**

a. 3–4 individuals
b. 5–7 individuals
c. 8–12 individuals
d. 13–20 individuals

**24. If the schedule performance index of a project is 93% and the cost performance index is 105%, this means that the project is:**

a. ahead of schedule and over budget
b. ahead of schedule and under budget
c. behind schedule and over budget
d. behind schedule and under budget

**25. According to Ludwig von Bertalanffy's general systems theory, the four elements in a system include input, processes, output, and:**

a. feedback
b. evaluation
c. remediation
d. authority

**26. If the NPD practitioner is asked to manage a project that is outside of that person's area of expertise, the best solution is to:**

a. refuse to manage the project
b. carry out intensive study in preparation
c. use consultants
d. hire additional staff

**27. According to the American Nurses Association (ANA), a healthy work environment has three key elements: empowerment, satisfaction, and**

a. flexibility
b. safety
c. service
d. compensation

**28. Which situation best lends itself to the use of scripting to aid communication?**

a. Providing a painful treatment
b. Comforting a parent whose child is ill
c. Participating in a team meeting
d. Providing a patient with discharge instructions

**29. The first step in protecting sensitive information is to:**

a. determine where information is to be stored
b. assess the types of information safeguards that are currently in place
c. identify which information needs to be protected
d. develop a plan to safeguard sensitive information

**30. With remote learning, the biggest challenge is typically:**

a. maintaining the motivation to learn
b. using technology correctly
c. having an unreliable internet connection
d. dealing with distracting environments

**31. When developing an operational excellence strategy for a healthcare organization, it is generally best to:**

a. implement changes throughout the organization
b. focus only on major problem areas
c. develop champions of the changes
d. start small and build on successes

**32. Educational neuroscience refers to a theory about learning that includes the:**

a. brain and learned responses
b. mind, brain, and education
c. teacher, learner, and environment
d. mind, environment, and opportunities

**33. Which type of network is most commonly used by hospitals?**

a. PAN
b. WAN
c. LAN
d. MAN

**34. When providing feedback to a team, it is essential to:**

a. address all feedback to the team as a whole
b. provide individual feedback
c. avoid all specifics
d. address only positive observations

**35. C. When developing a strategic plan, the NPD practitioner should look at the future needs of the organization in:**

a. 2–4 years
b. 5–9 years
c. 10–15 years
d. 16–20 years

**36. When establishing a timeline for a project, the first step is to identify the:**

a. team members
b. list of tasks
c. anticipated completion date
d. dependencies

**37. The primary purpose of using barcode scanners in hospitals is to:**

a. save time
b. save money
c. provide data
d. reduce errors

**38. The primary principle to consider when selecting learning technology is to determine if the technology:**

a. is cost-effective
b. adds value
c. is scalable
d. is customizable

**39. According to Rita and Kenneth Dunn's learning styles model, five basic elements that affect learning include environmental, emotional, sociological, physical, and**

a. imaginative
b. educational
c. neurological
d. psychological

**40. During the accreditation process for the Joint Commission:**

a. surveyors randomly select patients to follow
b. the administration chooses patients for the surveyors
c. no patients are followed or interviewed
d. only historical, not current, patient records are surveyed

**41. If an individual is noncommittal, contributes little to a conversation, and is unwilling to take sides when a conflict or difference of opinion occurs, the communication style that the individual is using is:**

a. assertive communication
b. passive communication
c. aggressive communication
d. passive-aggressive communication

**42. With respect to hospital electronic health records, the Medicare Promoting Interoperability Program objectives include health information exchange, provider-to-patient exchange, public health and clinical data exchange, and:**

a. risk management
b. clinical decision support system
c. multifactor authentication
d. electronic prescribing

**43. The primary purpose of role clarification in a team is to:**

a. prevent conflict
b. control uncooperative members
c. improve functioning
d. establish leadership

**44. For American Nurses Credentialing Center (ANCC) NPD certification renewal, how many continuing education hours (CEHs) must be completed?**

a. 75
b. 50
c. 30
d. 15

**45. A mission statement of an organization should include:**

a. future goals rather than what has already been achieved
b. lists of achievable aims and anticipated outcomes
c. measurable steps taken to achieve goals
d. a reflection of the current status, its purpose, and its role

**46. Before instituting changes, the NPD practitioner identifies champions within the organization, expecting that they will:**

a. advocate for and promote change
b. become barriers to change
c. assist with the logistics of change
d. provide financial support

**47. If using Zoom or a similar application for virtual classes, and the audio and visual keep lagging, the initial troubleshooting should be to:**

a. check the service status
b. update the Zoom software
c. check the internet connection
d. restart the program

**48. According to Patricia Benner's stages of clinical competence (novice to expert), the "competent" stage requires:**

a. 1–2 years of experience
b. 2–3 years of experience
c. 3–4 years of experience
d. 4–5 years of experience

**49. When carrying out research, if the method of selecting subjects results in a cohort that is not representative of the target population, this is an example of:**

a. sampling bias
b. confirmation bias
c. nonresponse bias
d. information bias

**50. Which type of organizational culture is exemplified by a workplace in which people have valued skills that are easily transferable to other organizations?**

a. Stable learning
b. Group
c. Independent
d. Insecure

**51. Which of the following is a module included in the transition to practice model for newly licensed nurses?**

a. Quality improvement
b. Multidisciplinary collaboration
c. Compliance issues
d. Malpractice and negligence

**52. According to National Institute of Standards and Technology (NIST) guidelines, which one of the following password examples best meets current guidelines for passwords?**

a. m3d3c1n3
b. 12161982
c. Bowser$2
d. Goattreepencil

**53. If the NPD practitioner designs a new type of protective gear, the design can be protected through:**

a. trademark
b. patent
c. copyright
d. trade secret

**54. An effective strategy in committees to deal with "squashers," who are averse to any change and criticize all suggestions and possible solutions, is to:**

a. tell the individuals directly to stop criticizing others' suggestions
b. interrupt the individuals each time they make a negative comment
c. remove the individuals from the committee altogether
d. ask to hold all comments and criticisms until all suggestions are made

**55. For which of the following types of measurement data is there no measure of variability?**

a. Nominal
b. Ordinal
c. Interval
d. Ratio

**56. An important element of provision 1 of the ANA Code of Ethics for Nurses ("The nurse practices with compassion and respect for the inherent dignity, worth, and unique attributes of every person") is:**

a. assignment and delegation of nursing activities/tasks
b. professional boundaries
c. the right to self-determination
d. protection of the rights of privacy and confidentiality

**57. A committee comprising individuals and experts who guide a project through to completion is referred to as a:**

a. steering committee
b. ad hoc committee
c. standing committee
d. advisory committee

**58. Which of the following is a requirement for the ANCC Magnet Recognition Program?**

a. The chief nursing officer (CNO) must hold a minimum of a bachelor of science (BS) degree in nursing or an allied field
b. Nurse leaders must report directly to the CNO
c. 75% of nurse leaders must have a degree in nursing (BS or higher)
d. 100% of nurse managers must have a degree in nursing (BS or higher)

**59. If a nurse responds to the first workshop in a series by stating, "I didn't learn anything that I didn't already know; these workshops are a waste of time," this is an example of the logical fallacy of:**

a. missing the point
b. slippery slope
c. hasty generalization
d. false dichotomy

**60. According to Kurt Lewin and Edgar Schein's change theory, motivation to change (unfreezing) is characterized by:**

a. strong desire to change
b. survival anxiety and sometimes learning anxiety
c. needed changes are identified
d. new behavior that becomes habitual

**61. In order to develop continuing education courses for nurses in states in which continuing education is required, the continuing education provider must generally:**

a. apply to the state boards of nursing
b. notify the state boards of nursing
c. apply to a professional organization
d. develop and advertise courses

**62. The first stage in quantitative data analysis is to:**

a. describe the sample
b. prepare the data
c. test the measurement reliability
d. conduct exploratory analysis

**63. Which of the following is a characteristic of Lean Six Sigma?**

a. Focus on customer needs and complaints
b. Focus on quality rather than cost reduction
c. Short-term goals with strategies in place for up to 1 year
d. Performance improvement as the underlying belief system

**64. If a nurse is licensed and lives in an enhanced nursing license compact (eNLC) state but works in another eNLC state with a multistate license, and the state of residence requires 30 continuing education units (CEUs) for license renewal but the state of employment requires 10 CEUs, how many CEUs must the nurse complete?**

a. 10
b. 20
c. 30
d. 40

**65. When managing a project, the project manager should consider the three-sphere model for systems management, which includes business, technology, and**

a. administration
b. communication
c. production
d. organization

**66. When carrying out risk analysis for electronic protected health information (ePHI), the first step is:**

a. identification of threats
b. system characterization
c. control analysis
d. identification of vulnerabilities

**67. According to John Watson's theory of behaviorism, the response to negative behavior/outcomes should be to:**

a. ignore them
b. provide a positive response
c. provide a negative response
d. vary the response according to the individual

**68. Under the Health Insurance Portability and Accountability Act of 1996 (HIPAA) Privacy Rule, which of the following situations may be considered to be an episode of incidental disclosure and not a violation if overheard or observed by others?**

a. Mistaking a patient's friend for their spouse and giving information about treatment
b. Writing a patient's name and diagnosis on a public sign-in sheet
c. Discussion in the hospital cafeteria about a patient's condition
d. Discussion with a patient about laboratory reports in a joint treatment area

**69. The four requirements for a virtual reality experience include the virtual world, immersion into that world, interactivity, and:**

a. sensory feedback
b. scoring system
c. personal avatars
d. augmented reality

**70. Typically, if developing a 1 CEU course, the NPD practitioner would plan to provide content for:**

a. 1 contact hour
b. 5 contact hours
c. 10 contact hours
d. 15 contact hours

**71. The best measure of nurse satisfaction is:**

a. lack of complaints
b. low use of sick time
c. improved retention rates
d. decreased nursing errors

**72. The NPD practitioner is developing a continuing education course entitled "Informatics for nurses" and plans 60 minutes of lecture followed by 120 minutes of hands-on practice and 30 minutes of assessment. How many contact hours does this equal?**

a. 0.5
b. 1.0
c. 3.0
d. 3.5

**73. The HIPAA Security Rule requires three kinds of safeguards: administrative, physical, and**

a. technical
b. environmental
c. secure
d. personal

**74. According to Claude Shannon's information theory, when describing the sender–receiver feedback loop, the channel is the:**

a. sender
b. receiver
c. method of delivery
d. form that the message takes

**75. If a healthcare organization is using the safe harbor method of deidentifying sensitive information, which of the following must be removed?**

a. Picture of a nonfacial wound
b. Mother's maiden name
c. Year of birth
d. Diagnosis

**76. A written (document) or artistic work (painting, image) is under copyright protection:**

a. immediately after it is created in a tangible form
b. from the time a copyright registration is applied for
c. after the material is registered for copyright
d. after a search shows that the work is free of plagiarism

**77. Regarding the six Ss that comprise the 6S pyramid of evidence, which S forms the base?**

a. Systems
b. Summaries
c. Studies
d. Syntheses

**78. The most reliable method of conducting a patient satisfaction survey is with a:**

a. telephone survey
b. written survey
c. email survey
d. personal interview

**79. With smartphone ownership being ubiquitous among healthcare workers, it is important for a healthcare organization to:**

a. ban cellphones during clinical hours
b. allow only phones with encryption
c. require that all phones are registered with the organization
d. establish policies for cellphone use

**80. In order to be considered by the ANCC as a content expert, the nurse must spend what percentage of professional time engaged in work associated with the nurse's certification area?**

a. 25%
b. 50%
c. 75%
d. 100%

**81. A computer-based training course that is developed as part of an educational expansion project is referred to as a:**

a. deliverable
b. by-product
c. outcome
d. product

**82. Knowledge of which of the following is especially important for an individual who provides customer service?**

a. Cognitive development
b. Psychoanalytic theory
c. Anger management
d. Behavioral psychology

**83. When developing continuing education courses that involve the psychomotor domain of learning, such as computer skills, which of the following is most essential?**

a. Role playing and reflective exercises
b. Spaced lessons with reinforcement of learning
c. Time for repeated practice
d. Journal keeping

**84. If a hacker sends an email using the name of a person in the information technology (IT) department that requests information, such as a username and password, this is an example of:**

a. phishing
b. spoofing
c. RAT
d. cloaking

**85. The seven Cs of communication include clear, concise, concrete, correct, coherent, complete, and:**

a. compelling
b. courteous
c. careful
d. collaborative

**86. Continuing education aimed at the cognitive domain of learning is ordered according to complexity, with the least complex being:**

a. knowledge
b. application
c. synthesis
d. evaluation

**87. The most efficient way to develop computer-based learning modules is to:**

a. follow the format of in-person instruction
b. use a learning management system (LMS)
c. focus on the content
d. hire designers and subject matter experts

**88. If a nurse discusses a patient's care plan with the occupational therapist who is also caring for the patient to determine the best intervention, this is an example of:**

a. internal collaboration
b. external collaboration
c. community collaboration
d. strategic alliance

**89. Advancement through the clinical ladder should be based on:**

a. duration of employment
b. personal relationships
c. clinical skills
d. recommendations

**90. In negotiation, if one party concedes to the other but the losing side gains little or nothing, this approach is referred to as:**

a. compromise
b. avoidance
c. competition
d. accommodation

**91. Which one of the following statements is the best example of feedback for a simulation exercise?**

a. "You made a lot of errors in this simulation."
b. "You omitted the epinephrine, causing the subsequent problems."
c. "You need to do this simulation again."
d. "You seemed very flustered throughout the procedure."

**92. When sharing data, a standard deviation should always be reported along with the:**

a. mean
b. median
c. range
d. percentile

**93. Which of the following is a characteristic of adult learning according to Malcolm Knowles and the theory of andragogy?**

a. Team-directed
b. Theoretical
c. Flexibility
d. Relevancy-oriented

**94. The primary purpose of a digital dashboard is to:**

a. provide a snapshot of the status of a department or organization
b. alert staff to compliance issues and changes in procedures
c. remind staff of meetings and responsibilities
d. improve patient care and outcomes

**95. Which of the following is the first stage of situational awareness?**

a. Anticipation
b. Understanding information
c. Information gathering
d. Experience

**96. If the NPD practitioner designs an instructional module that involves role playing, at which domain of learning is this primarily aimed?**

a. Psychomotor
b. Cognitive
c. Psychomotor and affective
d. Affective

**97. If the NPD practitioner tracks trends in the organization's internal and external environments as part of the development of strategic plans, this is an example of:**

a. professional readiness
b. environmental scanning
c. needs assessment
d. auditing

**98. To prevent a newly hired nurse from feeling overwhelmed when orientation ends, orientation should include:**

a. ongoing mentoring
b. a period of job shadowing
c. incentive pay
d. flexible scheduling

**99. According to Patrick Lencioni's Five Behaviors pyramid profile system for effective teams, the base of the pyramid is:**

a. commitment
b. trust
c. accountability
d. conflict

**100. To help ensure effective virtual meetings, the first step should be to:**

a. establish rules/norms for the meetings
b. send out the agenda in advance
c. query participants regarding their preferences
d. allot each participant a set amount of time

**101. The elements of nursing care that are reflected by nursing-sensitive indicators include:**

a. input, throughput, and output
b. assessment, implementation, and evaluation
c. monitor, treat, and record
d. structure, process, and outcomes

**102. If the fiscal year (the budgetary year) at an organization coincides with that of the state legislature and the US Congress, the fiscal year would go from:**

a. January 1 to December 31
b. October 1 to September 30
c. July 1 to June 30
d. August 1 to July 31

**103. Which one of the following types of data provides the highest level of evidence?**

a. Cohort study
b. Meta-analysis
c. Case study
d. Randomized controlled trial

**104. After discharge or the last contact with an adult patient, a hospital must keep the patient's health records for:**

a. 2 years
b. 5 years
c. 10 years
d. varying times, depending on the state

**105. When carrying out evidence-based research, which type of sampling has the highest probability of bias?**

a. Purposive
b. Quota
c. Convenience
d. Snowball

**106. When developing in-service programs to address deficiencies in care or procedures, the usual place to begin is with:**

a. the nursing supervisors
b. the accreditation report
c. a staff survey
d. the board of directors' recommendations

**107. The most critical aspect of time management is:**

a. prioritization
b. consistency
c. flexibility
d. self-assessment

**108. The first (doing) stage of role transition usually occurs over a period of about:**

a. 1–2 months
b. 2–3 months
c. 3–4 months
d. 4–5 months

**109. When using John Kotter's eight-step change model to integrate findings of evidence-based research into practice, the first phase is to:**

a. establish urgency
b. develop a vision
c. empower action
d. create a coalition

**110. If using SWOT analysis as part of action planning, low rates of reimbursement would be classified under:**

a. internal environment: strengths
b. internal environment: weaknesses
c. external environment: opportunities
d. external environment: threats

**111. The four primary core criteria for credentialing and privileging are licensure, education, competence, and:**

a. years of experience
b. performance ability
c. observation
d. certifications

**112. With smart pumps, the most frequent errors are with:**

a. use of the drug library
b. secondary infusions
c. wrong patient
d. incorrect dosage input

**113. The first step in the educational planning process and assessment is generally to:**

a. collect data from multiple sources
b. carry out in-person observations
c. identify expected outcomes
d. review budgetary concerns

**114. If the operating budget for the department is reevaluated each budget period to determine if it should be partially or completed funded, this type of budget is referred to as:**

a. fixed
b. flexible
c. zero-based
d. rolling

**115. During the planning phase, when developing strategies for an education program, it is most important for the NPD practitioner to:**

a. outline the schedule of classes
b. ensure that the materials used are cost-effective
c. determine the best classroom environment
d. individualize the content to the target learners

**116. If the NPD practitioner wants to purchase a simulation mannequin for training purposes and the fiscal year starts July1, the budgetary planning should begin in:**

a. December
b. February
c. April
d. May

**117. Which type of validity describes the degree to which a researcher can determine that the independent variable produced a change in the dependent variable?**

a. Statistical conclusion validity
b. Construct validity
c. External validity
d. Internal validity

**118. During the implementation stage of an education plan, one of the primary roles of the NPD practitioner is to:**

a. consider the needs of adult learners
b. coordinate various resources and systems
c. identify expected outcomes
d. use data to identify needs

**119. Which of the following is a team-based prospective analysis method that attempts to identify and correct failures in a process before its use to ensure positive outcomes?**

a. Five whys
b. Root cause analysis
c. Failure mode and effects analysis
d. Fault tree analysis

**120. When using PDSA (also referred to as the Deming cycle) for process improvement, during which phase is the action plan developed?**

a. P
b. D
c. S
d. A

**121. The most important factor in healthcare customer service is:**

a. prompt responses to complaints
b. good communication skills
c. excellence in healthcare
d. accessibility

**122. During the evaluation phase of the education design process, it is especially important for which of the following to be engaged in evaluation?**

a. The board of directors
b. Administrative staff
c. Consultants
d. Learners

**123. The initial strategy in developing a culture of empowerment is to:**

a. define responsibilities
b. outline expectations
c. reward innovations
d. identify key stakeholders

**124. For the Skills Base competency management model, the three necessary components are:**

a. ability, desire, and knowledge
b. time, training, and talent
c. affective, cognitive, and psychomotor
d. attitude, aptitude, and accomplishment

**125. Which of the following likely indicates a healthy work–life balance?**

a. Working for the salary that allows one to live the life they desire
b. Feeling that work is at the center of life
c. Volunteering to work overtime and on holidays
d. Leaving work on time and refusing overtime assignments

**126. The purpose of CMS core measures is to:**

a. ensure compliance with regulations
b. standardize procedures
c. produce better patient outcomes for common conditions
d. reduce the costs of care

**127. If the NPD practitioner asks learners to work together to develop a patient instruction pamphlet as part of a training series, this teaching model is referred to as:**

a. goal focused
b. project based
c. problem based
d. anchored

**128. According to the 10-20-30 rule for PowerPoint or other presentation software, the font size for the text should be:**

a. larger than 10 points
b. 10 to 20 points
c. smaller than 30 points
d. 30 points or larger

**129. Establishing a culture of safety within an organization requires an initial commitment from:**

a. leadership
b. staff members
c. community members
d. the board of directors

**130. To disseminate research findings to the broadest healthcare audience, the best method is generally:**

a. presentation at a professional organization conference
b. publication in the popular press
c. presentation in a journal club
d. publication in a professional journal

**131. An impact evaluation is intended to measure:**

a. the appropriateness of the teaching
b. whether the learners gained the intended knowledge
c. the program's effects on the organization or the greater community
d. whether the program attained the stated goals

**132. The five major functional areas in the hospital incident command system include administrative, logistics, planning, finance, and:**

a. hazards
b. operations
c. environment
d. communication

**133. When conducting a root cause analysis, it is especially important to:**

a. assign specific blame to an individual for an incident
b. include subjective and objective observations
c. prospectively analyze for further such events
d. identify contributing factors as well as the direct cause

**134. When preparing a formal report, a table of contents should be included for documents of more than:**

a. 5 pages
b. 7 pages
c. 10 pages
d. 12 pages

**135. If an analysis of data shows no outliers, the preferred statistic to report is the:**

a. median
b. mean
c. mode
d. range

**136. If an employer wants to ask whether a job applicant has a disability that requires accommodation, under the Americans with Disabilities Act, when can the employer do so?**

a. During the initial interview
b. After the person starts work
c. After hiring the person but before work starts
d. At any time

**137. In a just culture, if a nurse who has been caring for a patient for 3 days is observed greeting the patient by name and giving the patient a medication without checking the patient's identification band, an appropriate response would be:**

a. coaching the nurse and reviewing procedures
b. taking no action because the nurse knows the patient
c. suspending the nurse until remedial coursework is completed
d. recommending the release of the nurse for dangerous behavior

**138. The primary purpose of a process evaluation is to:**

a. determine if learners acquired the intended knowledge
b. justify expenditures for the program
c. determine if the teaching is appropriate
d. make necessary adjustments to the program

**139. Which generation is most likely to enjoy small talk as a way to build relationships and reach consensus and values working as part of a team?**

a. Silent generation (born 1927–1945)
b. Baby boomers (born 1946–1964)
c. Generation X (born 1960s–1980)
d. Generation Y/Millennials (born 1981–2000)

**140. When conducting a literature review in a database using the PICOT format, the C refers to:**

a. correlation
b. constraints
c. comparison/control
d. criteria

**141. The first step in carrying out a needs assessment is to determine the:**

a. available resources
b. target learners
c. time frame
d. outcome goals

**142. According to TJC, if a sentinel event occurs at a hospital, within how many business days must the hospital prepare a corrective action plan?**

a. 20
b. 30
c. 45
d. 60

**143. The least effective means of providing health information to a population with low health literacy is with:**

a. audiotapes
b. pictures and illustrations
c. videos
d. printed materials

**144. If using simulations in a lab as part of orientation of newly hired nurses, the learners should be:**

a. provided guidelines about specific objectives
b. expected to know appropriate interventions
c. asked to develop objectives as part of the simulation
d. guided step by step through the simulations

**145. If a researcher chooses a group of patients without disease, assesses risk factors, and then follows the group over time to determine which ones develop disease, this type of study is a:**

a. case control study
b. cross-sectional study
c. prospective cohort study
d. meta-analysis

**146. If a healthcare organization requires multiple orientation and continuing education courses for a wide range of staff in four different locations, the best method to manage this is likely:**

a. use an LMS
b. conduct all classes at one site
c. hire additional staff
d. conduct all classes via cloud-based video conferencing

**147. When developing a Gantt chart to set a timeline for program management, what type of dependency requires that the predecessor begins before the successor ends?**

a. Finish-to-finish
b. Start-to-start
c. Finish-to-start
d. Start-to-finish

**148. If, during a brainstorming session about quality improvement processes, the participants begin judging suggestions as they are contributed, the role of the NPD practitioner is to:**

a. encourage free expression of ideas and judgments
b. bring participants back to only expressing ideas first
c. outline the suggestions and the judgments
d. reprimand participants for being judgmental

**149.When carrying out evidence-based research and testing the reliability of instruments, the three important attributes include stability, equivalence, and:**

a. applicability
b. construct validity
c. external consistency
d. internal consistency

**150. Expenditures for advertising to promote a healthcare program are referred to as:**

a. variable costs
b. operating costs
c. sunk costs
d. direct costs

# Answer Key and Explanations

**1. C:** Implementation. Phases of the traditional project life cycle are as follows:

- Concept: Establishment of needs and work breakdown structure, preliminary estimate of costs.
- Development: More accurate estimate of costs, more detailed work breakdown structure.
- Implementation: Accurate estimate of costs, provision of performance reports to stakeholders.
- Close-out: Work completed, final report/documentation.

**2. B:** If a new type of electronic device is available for healthcare networks, the most important initial consideration for its purchase is device integration—that is, whether the device will connect to and function with existing hardware and software. Although software is usually available that can get a device to function, once it is in place, it can affect the entire network in unforeseen ways. Any new device needs to go through threat and vulnerability testing to ensure that it is working effectively and safely.

**3. C:** If the NPD practitioner is applying for a grant through the HRSA or other government agencies, the person should plan at least 40 hours to complete the application. For example, HRSA applications can be up to 80 pages in length and include sections on goals and objectives, needs, response and impact, resources and capabilities, and budget. Once an application is submitted, it can take up to 6 months before a decision is made about funding.

**4. A:** According to Meleis's transitions theory regarding change, transition conditions include facilitators and inhibitors; that is, one attaches perceptions about or meanings to health and illness or other experiences, and these perceptions can either facilitate or inhibit the ability of the individual to achieve a transition. Transitions usually involve a critical point or marker event that propels the individual to make a change. Process indicators and outcome indicators are used to assess progress toward the transition.

**5. B:** Leapfrog Hospital Safety Grade rankings provide a hospital report card that shows achievement toward standards in multiple areas including specific surgical procedures, such as total hip replacement and pancreatic resection for cancer. Areas covered in the ratings include preventing and responding to patient harm, medication safety, healthcare-associated infections, maternity care, pediatric care, critical care, complex adult and pediatric surgery, elective outpatient adult and pediatric surgery, and care for elective outpatient surgery patients.

**6. D:** Supervision. The five rights of delegation include:

1. Right task: An appropriate task to delegate for a specific individual.
2. Right circumstance: Considering the setting, resources, time factors, safety factors, and all other relevant factors to determine appropriateness.
3. Right person: By virtue of education/skills to perform a task for the right individual.
4. Right direction: Clear description of the task, the purpose, any limits, and expected outcomes.
5. Right supervision: Able to supervise, intervene as needed, and evaluate performance of the task.

**7. A:** When conducting a review of literature as part of research of best practices, the first thing to consider is the source of the material. Material from a juried journal, such as the *American Journal of Medicine* or the *American Journal of Nursing,* has more credibility compared to material from the popular press, such as *People* magazine. Next, review the author's credentials and check the date of publication and the date of the study to determine if the information is up to date. Then, identify the thesis or central claim, the organization and methodology, and review the evidence. Last, evaluate the overall article.

**8. C:** If using critical chain scheduling to ensure that a project with limited resources is completed on time, at the end of the project, it is necessary to include a project buffer. This is a time period planned after the work is completed but before the planned completion date in case there have been delays. Feedback buffers are also planned during the project before tasks on the critical chain that were preceded by noncritical tasks.

**9. B:** The type of conflict most often addressed in conflict-of-interest policies is financial. Conflict-of-interest policies should include a procedure for disclosure showing that a person's interests may be in conflict with those of the organization. The policy should apply to all individuals associated with an organization, including board members, administrators, consultants, committees, and medical staff as well as family members. Disclosure is typically done through a questionnaire that asks about the type of financial interests that may suggest a conflict of interest and affiliations with individuals or companies with which the organization does business.

**10. D:** The most effective way to monitor performance is through data collection. Monitoring begins with identifying performance measures and then determining how to measure the performance, analyzing the data, and comparing to internal and external data and benchmarks. This should lead to identification for improvement opportunities, supported by research and design or redesigns of processes and implementation of changes.

**11. A:** The first step in succession planning is to describe the behaviors, skills, and leadership qualities needed for the role. The next steps include outlining the needs of the organization and developing a formal written succession plan. An organization should have plans in place for emergency succession (usually with an internal candidate) and planned succession (with an internal or external candidate). Plans for succession should always be in place so that transitions are not disruptive to the organization. Planned succession may focus on internal and external candidates, depending on the needs of the organization.

**12. C:** According to the NPD Scope and Standards of Practice, for standard 1, "Assessment of practice gaps," one of the roles of the NPD practitioner is to analyze trends and supporting data. The NPD Scope and Standards of Practice includes standards of practice (which focus on the development of educational programs) and standards of professional performance (which include professional responsibilities, such as mentoring).

**13. D:** The primary focus in coaching should be on using questioning to help learners recognize problem areas. Coaching can include specific training, providing career information, and confronting issues of concern. Other effective methods of coaching include:

- Giving positive feedback, stressing what the learner is doing right.
- Providing demonstrations and opportunities for question/answer periods.
- Providing regular progress reports so the learner understands areas of concern.
- Assisting the learner to establish personal goals for improvement.
- Providing resources to help the learner master material.

**14. A:** A critical element of virtual learning is interactivity. Interactivity means that the learner responds in some way to the content, such as by answering a question or making a choice. Interactivity that requires some action, like making a choice onscreen, is more effective than presenting a question for contemplation. Without interactivity, learners tend to tune out after a time and miss content, especially with asynchronous learning in which there is no opportunity to communicate in real time with the instructor or other learners.

**15. B:** When developing a promotional strategy, the first step is to determine the organizational goals, which should relate to the vision and mission statements as well. Once it is clear what the organization wants to achieve, then it is important to determine the target audience and what they want or need. Then, the marketing channels should be identified—that is, the methods that will be used for the promotion, such as emails, social media, print advertising, commercials, or other methods, and their costs.

**16. C:** CMS requires that medical records pertaining to billed services for Medicare Parts A and B be maintained for 7 years from the date of service in order to prove medical necessity regarding orders, certifications, referrals, prescriptions, and billing requests for services, items, or prescription drugs. Seven years may be more or fewer years than are required by individual states for record storage. Required documentation may include physician orders, therapy notes, assessment notes, photographs, evaluations (face to face), and correspondence to or from the patient.

**17. D:** The relational database arranges data in rows and columns (tables). Relational databases have been in use for about 50 years and are reliable for structured data. The language that is commonly used with relational databases is Structured Query Language (SQL). SQL is a fourth-generation programming language that uses syntax similar to human language to access, manipulate, and retrieve data from relational database management systems.

**18. B:** If the NPD practitioner presents a potential decision but seeks input from staff or teams before making the final decision based on this input, that leadership style is characterized as participatory. Participatory leadership is time-consuming because the staff needs time to review the decision and provide input, and this approach to leadership may result in compromises that are not wholly satisfactory to management or staff. However, this process is motivating to staff who feel that their expertise and input are valued.

**19. C:** Notification to individuals must be made by mail (or email if permission has been given to do so) within 60 days. If unable to contact fewer than 10 individuals, alternate notification, such as by telephone, is permitted. However, for 10 or more individuals, notice must be placed on the organization's website for 90 days with a toll-free telephone number or notice provided in print or through broadcast media. Individual breaches of fewer than 500 individuals are reported annualy to the Department of Health and Human Services secretary, whereas breaches of 500 or more individuals require that the secretary be notified within 60 days.

**20. A:** According to Bandura's theory of social learning, human behavior is learned through observation and modeling. The four conditions that Bandura proposed for modeling include:

1. Attention: The degree of attention paid to modeling can depend on many variables (physical, social, or environmental).
2. Retention: People's ability to retain models depends on symbolic coding, creating mental images, organizing thoughts, and rehearsing (mentally or physically).

3. Reproduction: The ability to reproduce a model depends on physical and mental capabilities.
4. Motivation: Motivation may derive from past performance, rewards, or vicarious modeling.

**21. D:** Risk management's primary responsibility toward incident reports is to review the reports to identify possible failures in the system. Studies show that errors are grossly underreported; however, increasingly, incident reports are generated by electronic data that indicate an error has occurred, such as in medication administration. Incident report reviews are less comprehensive and time-consuming and more cost-effective than retrospective medical record reviews but can yield valuable information, so providing staff with incentives for reporting incidents and confidentiality is important.

**22. B:** The primary purpose of multifactor authentication is to prevent data breaches. Passwords are fairly easy to uncover, so using multifactor authentication adds another step to data access and gives protection against hackers. After inputting the password, one or more additional authentications are required, such as the use of a token or other identification device and sometimes biometric authentication, such as a fingerprint or iris scan, as well.

**23. C:** Focus groups usually comprise 8–12 members. A smaller number may lack adequate diversity, whereas a larger number may make it too difficult for the group members to stay focused. The group usually meets for approximately 1.5–2 hours for a focused discussion on a particular topic led by a facilitator or moderator with a recorder present and sometimes behind a one-way mirror. A transcript of the meeting should be prepared for study. Nontraditional focus groups are sometimes conducted by telephone conference calls, internet groups, or videoconferences.

**24. D:** If the schedule performance index of a project is 93% and the cost performance index is 105%, this means that the project is behind schedule and under budget. For the schedule performance index, less than 100% is behind schedule and more than 100% is ahead of schedule. For the cost performance index, at 100%, planned and actual costs are equal; and, at more than 100%, the project is under budget. At less than 100%, it is over budget.

**25. A:** According to von Bertalanffy's general systems theory, the four elements in a system include:

1. Input: This is what goes into a system in terms of energy or materials.
2. Processes: These are the actions that take place in order to transform input.
3. Output: This is the result of the interrelationship between input and processes.
4. Feedback: This is information that can be used for evaluation and correction of the system.

According to this theory, a change in any element in a system will impact the other elements and alter the outcomes, so systems must be viewed holistically.

**26. C:** If the NPD practitioner is asked to manage a project that is outside of that person's area of expertise, the best solution is to use consultants. When managing projects, it is common to need outside consultants with expertise in particular areas to ensure that no important details are overlooked and to more accurately identify necessary tasks and ensure the appropriate and desired outcomes. Average hourly wages for consultants vary but are usually less than $100 per hour, although this depends on the area of expertise.

**27. B:** According to the ANA, a healthy work environment has three key elements:

1. Empowerment: Autonomy commensurate with position and training and participation in decision making through some type of shared governance.
2. Satisfaction: Adequate wages, reasonable workload, good scheduling of work hours, flexible working schedules, and a supportive and nonpunitive environment.
3. Safety: Environmental safety (fire escapes, good air quality, and adequate lighting and heating); physical safety; and freedom from bullying, violence, and physical and emotional abuse.

**28. D:** The situation that best lends itself to the use of scripting to aid in communication is providing a patient with discharge instructions. Scripting does not mean memorizing specific words to say; rather, it means knowing in advance what issues to address, such as wound care, medications, and return visits, and having an idea of how to address those issues (e.g., by stating "Mrs. Smith, let's talk first about your wound care"). It is more difficult to prepare in advance for emotional situations because they vary widely and responses cannot always be anticipated.

**29. C:** The first step in protecting sensitive information is to identify which information needs to be protected followed by where and how the data are stored and the types of safeguards that are currently in place. Then, a comprehensive plan must be developed to protect sensitive information, to include names and contact information (addresses, telephone numbers), characteristics (age, marital status, religion, gender), personally identifiable information (social security number, ID number, driving license number, mother's maiden name, credit/criminal history), financial data (credit cards, bank account numbers, personal identification numbers, security codes), health information, insurance information, and employment status.

**30. A:** With remote learning, the biggest challenge is typically maintaining the motivation to learn. Learners often start out enthusiastically but lose focus and become bored, especially if the remote learning is asynchronous and lacks interactivity. Other problems include the instructors' and the learners' inability to use the technology correctly, especially those with little computer literacy. In some places, an unreliable internet connection can interfere with remote learning, and dealing with distracting environments (children, background noise) can interfere with learning.

**31. D:** When developing an operational excellence strategy for a healthcare organization, it is generally best to start small and build on successes—for example, a unit may institute the use of a checklist for specific procedures or the emergency department may focus on reducing wait times. Once staff members see concrete evidence that changes have a positive effect on outcomes, they are typically more willing to make the necessary changes and to help identify any needed changes.

**32. B:** Educational neuroscience refers to a theory about learning that includes the mind, brain, and education. According to this view of learning, research in the fields of psychology and neuroscience should be used in the field of education in a collaborative effort because it provides insight into the way people learn and integrate knowledge. Brain imaging techniques, such as magnetic resonance imaging, have provided information about how the brain processes information. Educational neuroscience emphasizes the need for transdisciplinary collaboration.

**33. C:** A local area network (LAN) is most commonly used by hospitals. The LAN connects computers in a relatively small area, such as a building. This allows data to be transmitted quickly and with a high degree of security. A personal area network (PAN) connects devices (usually wirelessly) to a range of about 30 feet. A metropolitan area network (MAN) connects computers in geographic areas, such as a city, through an interconnection of LANs. The wide area network (WAN) connects computer systems over large areas, such as states or even different countries, through various means (satellite links, cables, telephone).

**34. A:** When providing feedback to a team, it is essential to address all feedback to the team as a whole rather than providing individual feedback because individual feedback should always be done one-on-one in private—for example, when providing feedback to a group, one can focus on how the group members worked together and divided tasks or how they missed opportunities to collaborate. Feedback should include positive and negative observations. Feedback should be given immediately after an observation, if possible.

**35. C:** When developing a strategic plan, the NPD practitioner should look at the future needs of the organization in 10–15 years. Although establishing goals for the near future (2–4 years) is also important, strategic planning must look at extended periods. Periods beyond 15 years are difficult to plan for because of unforeseen changes in demographics and technology that may affect the needs of the organization.

**36. B:** When establishing a timeline for a project, the first step is to identify the list of tasks that must be completed followed by the duration of each task and the date by which they should be completed. Next, dependencies (something that has a relationship to another action) must be identified along with constraints, such as time, cost, and the scope of the project. The anticipated completion date is identified last because it is dependent on the other elements.

**37. D:** The primary purpose of using barcode scanners in hospitals is to reduce errors. For example, if a patient is given a wristband with a barcode, and all medications and treatments issued for the patient have the same barcode, the nurse must scan the barcode on the medication and the patient to ensure that they match. If they do, then the medication is automatically recorded in the patient's electronic health record. Barcodes and scanners are also commonly used for inventory control.

**38. B:** The primary principle to consider when selecting learning technology is to determine if the technology adds value to the learning process; that is, the technology should be better than what is currently available, should contribute in some way to a better learning experience for the learner, and should improve the quality of the education. The added value should be outlined as part of the justification for the purchase of new hardware or software.

**39. D:** According to Dunn and Dunn's learning styles model, five basic elements that affect learning include:

1. Environmental: Sound, light, temperature, and design.
2. Emotional: Motivation, persistence, responsibility, and structure.
3. Sociological patterns: Learning alone, the presence of an authority figure, and flexible learners.
4. Physical: Perceptual strengths (aural, visual, read/write, or kinesthetic), intake (food, drinks), time of day (morning learners, afternoon learners, and evening learners), and mobility (preference for sitting or moving around).
5. Psychological: Global (overview) versus analytic (step-by-step), hemispheric preference (right brain versus left brain), and impulsivity versus reflectivity.

**40. A:** During the TJC accreditation process, surveyors randomly select patients to follow and use their health records to trace their experiences in the healthcare organization. Surveyors make observations and carry out interviews with all levels of staff who interact with the selected patients. An organization seeking accreditation must first contact TJC about eligibility and must complete a detailed application.

**41. B:** If an individual is noncommittal, contributes little to a conversation, and is unwilling to take sides when a conflict or difference of opinion occurs, the communication style that the individual is using is passive communication. The person may avoid direct eye contact and appear nervous and fidgety if confronted. The individual may also show signs of anxiety, such as wringing the hands or crossing the arms. The passive communicator may respond inappropriately when angry, such as by laughing, and may believe that disagreeing with another person will be upsetting to that person or result in conflict, which the person wants to avoid.

**42. D:** With respect to hospital electronic health records, the Medicare Promoting Interoperability Program objectives include the following with points awarded for achieving each objective:

- Electronic prescribing: 10 points and 10 bonus points for query of a prescription drug monitoring program.
- Health information exchange: Send (20 points) and receive (20 points) health information.
- Provider-to-patient exchange: 40 points.
- Public health and clinical data exchange: Immunization registry and electronic case reporting (10 points) and public health registry, clinical data registry or syndromic surveillance reporting (5 bonus points).

**43. C:** The primary purpose of role clarification in a team is to improve functioning. The steps to role clarification include (1) write a role description, (2) write comments/advice on each other's role descriptions, (3) share descriptions and comments/advice, (4) provide feedback to each other regarding what the other person should do, (5) review and summarize the comments/advice, (6) negotiate what can and cannot be done, and (7) document agreements.

**44. A:** For ANCC certification renewal, 75 CEHs must be completed in addition to at least one of the other ANCC renewal categories in the specialty area of the certification. Renewal categories include (1) CEHs, (2) academic credits, (3) presentations, (4) evidence-based practice, quality improvement project, publication, or research, (5) preceptor hours, (6) professional service, (7) practice hours, and (8) assessment (if available).

**45. D:** The mission statement of an organization should include a reflection of the current status, its purpose, and its role. The mission statement should identify the organization or program, state its function, and outline the purpose and strategy of the organization or program. The mission statement should also reflect the vision statement, which reflects where the organization sees itself in the future, and it may include a detailed explanation with statements of the organizational values, philosophy, and history. Goals and objectives should be developed in support of the vision and mission statements.

**46. A:** Before instituting changes, the NPD practitioner identifies champions within the organization, expecting that they will advocate for and promote change. Staff are often resistant to change, sometimes expecting that change will result in more work, so identifying positive voices to counter the negative ones can help to facilitate change. In some cases, champions are part of the leadership, but champions can be found at all levels of an organization, and people may respond better to peers.

**47. C:** If using Zoom or a similar application for virtual classes, and the audio and visual keep lagging, the initial troubleshooting step should be to check the internet connection because this is generally where the problem lies. In some cases, a drain on the internet connection may be occurring from background downloads or concurrent streaming from a computer somewhere in the same network. It is important to keep the software updated, and Zoom, like other similar companies, sends update reminders.

**48. B:** According to Benner's stages of clinical competence, the competent stage requires 2–3 years of experience. The nurse at this stage has some mastery of new situations and goals and can cope well but may require time for planning and may lack flexibility. The five stages that Benner outlines include: novice (little experience, rule dependent), advanced beginner (some experience coping with new situations and formulating action plans), competent (able to function independently), proficient (looks at situations holistically), and expert (able to provide intuitive care based on much experience).

**49. A:** When carrying out research, if the method of selecting subjects results in a cohort that is not representative of the target population, this is an example of sampling (or selection) bias. For example, if all patients who develop urinary infections are evaluated per urine culture and sensitivities for microbial resistance, but only those patients with clinically evident infections are included, a number of patients with subclinical infections may be missed, skewing the results. Sampling/Selection bias is only a concern when participants in studies are specifically chosen for a study.

**50. C:** Independent. Organizational culture involves shared assumptions about behavior and working together in an organization. Basic types of organizational cultures include:

- Stable learning cultures in which people exercise skills and advance over time.
- Independent cultures in which people have valued skills that are easily transferable to other organizations.
- Group cultures in which there is strong identification and an emphasis on seniority.
- Insecure cultures with frequent staff layoffs and reorganization.

**51. A:** The transition to practice model for newly licensed nurses includes five modules:

1. Communication and teamwork.
2. Patient-centered care.
3. Evidence-based practice.
4. Quality improvement.
5. Informatics.

According to this model, the newly licensed nurse should learn through experiential practice. This model provides training for preceptors and requires preceptors to help guide newly hired nurses. The modules are available online for study.

**52. D:** According to NIST guidelines, the recommended password type example is Goattreepencil because these are three unrelated words that are easy for the user to remember but difficult to uncover, and the password is at least eight characters in length. NIST no longer recommends routinely changing passwords or the use of complex passwords with symbols because they are difficult to remember. Anniversary dates or birthdates, such as 12161982, should be avoided as should names of pets or children. Passwords that are easily deciphered, such as m3d3c1n3 (i.e., "medicine"), are not safe.

**53. B:** If the NPD practitioner designs a new type of protective gear, the design can be protected through a patent. Most patents last for 20 years after the date of filing. Copyright, on the other hand, typically lasts for 70 years. There are many different avenues used to protect intellectual property, depending on the type of property, including trademarks, patent, copyright, industrial design, trade secrets, database, and unfair competition.

**54. D:** An effective strategy in committees to deal with squashers, who are averse to any change and criticize all suggestions and possible solutions, is to begin the meeting by telling members to hold all comments and criticisms until all suggestions are made. This may require repeatedly reminding people to hold comments until a new pattern of behavior is established, but meetings will be more productive with members being less afraid to contribute.

**55. A:** There is no measure of variability with nominal data because the data form mutually exclusive sets, such as gender or ethnic background. Other forms of measurement data have measures of variability. Ordinal data can be ranked, such as from most effective to least effective. Interval data have no true zero, but results have equal intervals, such as temperature. Ratio data are similar to interval data but have a true zero point, such as age or height data.

**56. C:** An important element of provision 1 of the ANA Code of Ethics for Nurses ("The nurse practices with compassion and respect for the inherent dignity, worth, and unique attributes of every person") is the right to self-determination. Patients have the right to make decisions about their care, including the right to refuse care, and to receive information that is accurate and understandable. Nurses have the responsibility to be aware of patients' rights and to support their autonomy.

**57. A:** A committee comprising individuals and experts who guide a project through to completion is referred to as a steering committee. Other committee types include:

- Ad hoc: A temporary committee with a specific task to complete.
- Standing: Permanent committees with specific responsibilities, including general oversight of an organization.
- Advisory: Committee comprised of nonboard members and community members used to provide expert opinions.

**58. D:** A requirement for the ANCC Magnet Recognition Program is that 100% of nurse managers must have a degree in nursing (BS or higher). The CNO requires a minimum of a master of science (MS) degree. All nurse managers and nurse leaders must have a minimum of a BS or a graduate degree in nursing. Nurse leaders may or may not report directly to the CNO. Policies and procedures must be in place to allow and encourage confidential expressions of concern, and the organization must be in compliance with all federal compliance measures.

**59. C:** If a nurse responds to the first workshop in a series by stating, "I didn't learn anything that I didn't already know; these workshops are a waste of time," this is an example of the logical fallacy of hasty generalization. The nurse has made a judgment about the entire series based on too little information (the first workshop). Although it is illogical, this is a common reaction, so the first encounter that learners have is especially important in establishing their perceptions.

**60. B:** According to Lewin and Schein's change theory, motivation to change (unfreezing) is characterized by survival anxiety as previous beliefs are questioned and sometimes by learning anxiety, which may lead to resistance. The next step is the desire to change (unfrozen), during which dissatisfaction is strong enough to override defensive actions and the desire for change is strong but must be accompanied by identification of needed changes. The last stage is development of permanent changes (refreezing), during which the new behavior becomes habitual.

**61. A:** Although state boards of nursing vary in their requirements for continuing education and their requirements for continuing education providers, generally, in order to develop continuing education courses for nurses, the continuing education provider must apply to the state boards of nursing and meet the requirements outlined by the boards. The provider is granted a provider number, which must be present on the learner's certificate of completion. If a continuing education course is provided in house for purposes of employment rather than licensure, then application to the state board of nursing is not necessary.

**62. B:** The first stage in quantitative data analysis is to prepare the data so that they can be analyzed efficiently. The next step is to describe the sample and then test measurement reliability, followed by exploratory and confirmatory data analysis and post hoc analysis. Quantitative data analysis looks at objective or hard data and is often used to disseminate information obtained from surveys, questionnaires, or polls because the results quantify; that is, they show how much or how many.

**63. D:** Lean Six Sigma is a method that combines Six Sigma with concepts of "lean" thinking and focuses process improvement on strategic goals rather than on a project-by-project basis. Four characteristics of Lean Six Sigma include:

1. Performance improvement as the underlying belief system.
2. Long-term goals with strategies in place for 1- to 3-year periods.
3. Cost reduction through quality increases, supported by statistics evaluating the cost of inefficiencies.
4. Incorporation of an improvement methodology, such as define, measure, analyze, improve, and control; plan, do, check, and act; or other methods.

**64. C:** If a nurse is licensed and lives in an eNLC state but works in another eNLC state with a multistate license, and the state of residence requires 30 CEUs for license renewal but the state of employment requires 10, the nurse must complete 30 CEUs to meet the requirements of the state of residence. If the state of employment requires specific CEUs, the organization for which the nurse works may require that the nurse complete those CEUs.

**65. D:** When managing a project, the project manager should consider the three-sphere model for systems management, which includes:

1. Business: Cost-effectiveness/cost–benefit concerns, unexpected issues.
2. Technology: Considerations of the hardware and software needed, interoperability concerns, staff technological competency.
3. Organization: Who will be affected, what training will be needed, how will the training be supported, how to deal with unexpected issues.

**66. B:** When carrying out risk analysis for ePHI, the first step is system characterization. This includes a review of all hardware and software and support systems as well as a determination as to who "owns" or controls the applications; for example, the pharmacy may have one application that contains ePHI, and the laboratory may have a different application. Once the system has been reviewed and outlined, then threats to the system (internal, external, medical identity, breaches, red flags) and vulnerabilities should be identified. Control analysis reviews how the system deals with threats and vulnerabilities.

**67. A:** According to Watson's theory of behaviorism, the response to negative behavior/outcomes should be to ignore them. Watson believed that people could be completely controlled by proper application of reward. Thus, individuals are rewarded through praise or concrete rewards (points, prizes, computer time, salary increases, recognition) when they successfully carry out a particular behavior. While using positive reinforcement, negative reinforcement should be avoided because people may respond equally to both. When possible, negative outcomes should be ignored with responses given only to positive outcomes.

**68. D:** Under HIPAA's Privacy Rule, a discussion with a patient about laboratory reports in a joint treatment area may be considered to be an episode of incidental disclosure and not a violation if overheard or observed by others. Covered entities must use "reasonable safeguards" to prevent disclosure of the following:

- Discussions about coordinating care at nurse stations.
- Discussions about patient's condition with the patient, healthcare provider, or family member.
- Physician discussions with a patient regarding their condition in a semiprivate room.
- Training round discussions regarding a patient's condition in academic/training situations.
- Pharmacist discussion with a patient or physician over the phone or with a patient over the pharmacy counter.

**69. A:** The four requirements for a virtual reality experience include the virtual world, immersion into that world, interactivity, and sensory feedback. For example, exergames (games that involve exercise) are available to promote exercise such as golfing. The person moves the arms to simulate a stroke in a world that appears as a golf course. The person can move about that world and interact with the ball, receiving sensory feedback that includes seeing the golf ball fly in response to hitting it and hearing the sound of the ball's impact. Some virtual games include haptic feedback such as vibrations.

**70. C:** Typically, if developing a 1 CEU course, the NPD practitioner would plan to provide content for 10 contact hours with each contact hour lasting 50 to 60 minutes. Continuing education courses may be required for licensure/relicensure, employment, professional advancement, and certification/recertification. Continuing education requirements vary widely from one state to another, ranging from 0 to 45 every 2–3 years.

**71. C:** The best measure of nurse satisfaction is improved retention rates. The national turnover rate for nurses is approximately 19% a year, and each nurse that leaves employment costs the organization approximately $40,000. Coupled with the shortage of nurses, a high turnover rate can be costly to an organization and impact the quality of care, so investing in strategies to improve nurse satisfaction, such as flexible hours, shared governance, advancement, and tuition assistance, may save money over time.

**72. D:** If the NPD practitioner is developing a continuing education course entitled "Informatics for nurses" and plans 60 minutes of lecture followed by 120 minutes of hands-on practice and 30 minutes of assessment, this is equal to 3.5 contact hours. Calculation:

- 60 + 120 + 30 = 210.
- 210 ÷ 60 = 3.5.

**73. A:** The HIPAA Security Rule requires three kinds of safeguards:

1. Administrative: Policies and procedures, designation of privacy officer, training programs, risk management programs.
2. Physical: Locked doors, controlled access to equipment, appropriate placement of workstations and computer monitors.
3. Technical: End-to-end data encryption, passwords, authentication, secure data centers.

**74. C:** According to Shannon's information theory, when describing the sender–receiver feedback loop, the channel is the method of delivery. The communication process begins with the sender (the encoder) who determines the content of the message. The medium is the form that the message takes (digital, written, or audiovisual), and the channel is the method of delivery (mail, radio, TV, phone, or email). The recipient (receiver) who acts as the decoder determines the meaning from the message. Feedback helps to determine whether or not the communication is successful.

**75. B:** Mother's maiden name. The HIPAA Privacy Rule provides two methods of deidentification:

1. Expert determination (based on applying statistical or scientific principles): The expert must have appropriate knowledge and must document the method and analysis results.
2. Safe harbor deidentification removes 18 types of identifiers including name, geographic information, zip code, telephone number, license number, account number, mother's maiden name, FAX number, serial number of devices, email address, URLs, full-face photographs, all elements of dates (except the year), and biometric identifiers.

**76. A:** A written (document) or artistic work (paintings, images) is under copyright protection immediately after it is created in tangible form, such as a digital, video, or audio file or on paper. Ideas that have not yet been recorded in some tangible form cannot be copyrighted. Registering a copyright is not required but is an option and is necessary if the author should want to bring a plagiarism or improper use lawsuit at some later date. Sending a copy of a written work to oneself does not provide protection of copyright under the law, contrary to popular belief.

**77. C:** Regarding the six Ss that comprise the 6S pyramid of evidence, studies form the base. With evidence-based research, the individual will usually start at the top of the pyramid and work down toward the base when attempting to find information to support treatment approaches. The levels from top to bottom are as follows: systems, summaries, synopses of syntheses, syntheses, synopses of single studies, and single studies. Systems includes an electronic health record with a computerized decision support system that allows easy access to information.

**78. B:** The most relieable method of conductiong a patient satisfaction survey is with a written survey. Telephone calls are often screened, so response rates are low, and email surveys are easily ignored. Personal interviews are time- and cost-intensive. Patients should be provided written surveys at the end of care and should be encouraged to fill them out before leaving or as soon as possible. Compliance is better if surveys are short (10 or fewer questions) and to the point and if they allow for anonymous input.

**79. D:** With smartphone ownership being ubiquitous among healthcare workers, it is important for a healthcare organization to establish policies for smartphone use. This may include limiting personal calls to break times only and delineating how smartphones can be used as part of patient care, such as by accessing databases for information about a disorder. Policies should include consequences for misuse, the need for encryption when transmitting any PHI, etiquette for use including explaining to patients why information is being accessed, and avoiding smartphone distractions during on-duty work hours.

**80. B:** In order to be considered by ANCC as a content expert, the nurse must spend at least 50% of their professional time engaged in work associated with their certification area. Additionally, the nurse's certification must be current and active and the nurse's nursing license must be unencumbered by the state in which the nurse is licensed. The nurse must be willing to sign a volunteer agreement with ANCC and a conflict-of-interest form. The decision about inclusion is made by an appointments committee.

**81. A:** A computer-based training course (or any type of product) that is developed as part of an educational expansion project is referred to as a deliverable. The deliverable is an output (tangible or intangible) or a completed objective of the project. Deliverables may be internal (such as completion of assigned tasks) or external (such as a computer-based training course or periodic reports). Expected deliverables should be outlined at the beginning of a project.

**82. D:** Knowledge of behavioral psychology is especially important for an individual who provides customer service. Customer service requires a good understanding of behavior and emotional responses and methods of communication that can redirect anger and frustration. The individual in customer service must be an active listener and should be able to establish a sense of trust by being open and honest in all forms of communication, which may be face to face or via telephone, email, chat, or text messaging. Those in customer service need strong skills in communication, writing, and grammar.

**83. C:** When developing continuing education courses that involve the psychomotor domain of learning, such as computer skills, time for repeated practice is most essential. The psychomotor domain of learning, also known as the skills domain, focuses on fine and gross motor abilities required to carry out tasks. Teaching strategies for the psychomotor domain should focus on mastery of a skill rather than the cognitive and affective domains because psychomotor skills require singular attention.

**84. A:** If a hacker sends an email using the name of a person in the IT department that requests information, such as a username and password, this is an example of phishing. Hackers trick people into inadvertently providing information that will allow the hacker access to computer data. Spoofing is similar, but the person creates fake headers or even websites that look like authentic ones in order to obtain information. RAT (remote access tools) is a type of malware that allows a hacker to control the system on which it is installed. Cloaking is giving a false appearance. For example, malware may appear as a gaming application.

**85. B:** Courteous. The seven Cs of communication include:

1. Clear: Purpose in writing is clearly stated.
2. Concise: Be brief and direct.
3. Concrete: Provide details and factual information.
4. Correct: Stated grammatically and without errors.
5. Coherent: Stated logically.
6. Complete: All points are included.
7. Courteous: Friendly, persuasive.

**86. A:** Continuing education aimed at the cognitive domain of learning (also known as the thinking domain) is ordered according to complexity, with the least complex domain being knowledge. The order of domains in increasing complexity is as follows: knowledge, comprehension, application, analysis, synthesis, and evaluation. Studies show that for learning in the cognitive domain, distributed practice/education results in better retention than massed practice; therefore, lessons must be spaced appropriately and reinforcement should be planned for maximum retention. Much of traditional education is focused toward the cognitive domain of learning. Techniques used to develop cognitive abilities include lecture, one-on-one instruction, and computer-assisted instruction.

**87. B:** The most efficient way to develop computer-based learning modules is to use an LMS because the necessary software is built into the system, making the creation of content and embedding of audio and video files relatively straightforward. An LMS allows for easy testing and feedback and access to individual and aggregate data. It is important to focus on the learners and their needs and to recognize that a computer-based approach is different from in-person instruction.

**88. A:** If a nurse discusses a patient's care plan with the occupational therapist, who is also caring for the patient, to determine the best intervention, this is an example of internal collaboration, which is most often carried out face to face—although in a large organization, telephone, email, or text messaging may also be used. Internal collaboration takes place within an organization or program and may be formal, such as in team meetings, or informal, such as in conversations. External collaboration is often more formal and involves collaboration with those outside the organization and is often brought about by alliances, partnerships, and joint ventures.

**89. C:** Clinical ladder advancement should be based on the following:

- Clinical skills: Experience, certification in particular skills training (such as insertion of a peripherally inserted central catheter line).
- Leadership skills: Participation in shared governance, committees, mentoring, coaching, supervision.
- Education: Advanced degrees, national certification, continuing education courses, special training.
- Research: Participation in a journal club, clinical research, presentations, publications.
- Professional development: Participation in professional organizations, attending conferences, giving presentations.

**90. D:** Accommodation.

| **Approaches to negotiation** | |
|---|---|
| **Competition** | One party wins, and the other party loses. To prevail, one party must remain firm, but this can result in conflict. |
| **Accommodation** | One party concedes to the other, but the losing side may gain little or nothing. |
| **Avoidance** | When both parties dislike conflict, they may put off negotiating and nothing gets resolved, so the problems remain. |
| **Compromise** | Both parties make concessions in order to reach consensus, but this can result in decisions that suit no one. |
| **Collaboration** | Both parties get what they want, often through creative solutions. |

**91. B:** Feedback should be as objective as possible (e.g., "You omitted the epinephrine, causing the subsequent problems") so the learner has a clear idea of what went well and what did not.

Describing the learner's emotional status ("very flustered") provides no useful information for improvement. Vague statements ("a lot of errors") do not help the learner know what needs to be corrected. Doing the simulation again without knowing what went wrong may produce the same results.

**92. A:** When sharing data, the standard deviation should always be reported along with the mean because the standard deviation shows the average deviation from the mean in a data set. The standard deviation is plotted on the normal bell curve and shows how the data spread out from the mean. Usually, 68% of the data fall within one standard deviation of the mean and 95% within two deviations.

**93. D:** According to Knowles and the theory of andragogy, the characteristics of adult learning include:

- Practical and goal oriented: Provide overviews, summaries, examples, problem-solving exercises.
- Self-directed: Encourage active involvement and allow different options and responsibilities.
- Knowledgeable: Validate life experience/education and relate new material to that already mastered.
- Relevancy-oriented: Explain how information will be applied.
- Motivated: Provide certificates of achievement, recognition for achievements.

**94. A:** The primary purpose of a digital dashboard is to provide a snapshot of the status of a department or organization. The digital dashboard is a computer application that integrates a variety of performance measures or key indicators into one display (usually with graphs or charts) that provides an overview of an organization. Data may include the results of patient satisfaction surveys, infection rates, financial status, or any other measurement that is important to assess for its performance. Digital dashboards should be updated on a regular basis: daily, weekly, or monthly.

**95. C:** There are three stages to situational awareness:

1. Information gathering: Surveying the environment, being alert to any hazards or signs of danger, and gathering information from others who are present or have knowledge about the situation.
2. Understanding information: Processing the information and reaching conclusions based on that information.
3. Anticipation: Reaching conclusions about how the situation will affect the future status and instituting readiness actions.

**96. D:** If the NPD practitioner designs an instructional module that involves role playing, this is primarily aimed at the affective domain of learning. The affective domain of learning, also known as the feeling domain, relates to the emotional response that the learner has to learning rather than cognitive abilities; it cannot be adequately measured but only inferred. The five levels of affective behavior are receiving, responding, valuing, organizing, and characterizing. Teaching strategies include activities such as role-playing, gaming, and simulations, followed by debriefing or reflective exercises.

**97. B:** If the NPD practitioner tracks trends in the organization's internal and external environment as part of the development of strategic plans, this is an example of environmental scanning. Internal issues may include leadership changes, budgeting, staffing issues, and census. External issues may include demographics, technology, research, political issues, and economics. Many different factors may influence an organization.

**98. A:** To prevent a newly hired nurses from feeling overwhelmed when orientation ends, orientation should include ongoing mentoring. This provides support and gives the nurse the opportunity to benefit and learn from the expertise of others. Formal mentoring programs usually establish one-on-one mentoring relationships rather than the more informal mentoring that occurs when one nurse assists another. Many orientation programs are limited to a review of policies, procedures, and equipment with little preparation for the actual job functions.

**99. B:** According to Lencioni's Five Behaviors pyramid profile system for effective teams, the base of the pyramid is trust. Without trust, it is almost impossible to make progress. This pyramid is in response to Lencioni's Five Dysfunctions of teams:

1. Absence of trust.
2. Fear of conflict.
3. Lack of commitment.
4. Avoidance of accountability.
5. Inattention to results.

**100. A:** To help ensure effective virtual meetings, the first step should be to establish rules/norms for the meetings—for example, if there is a large group, participants may be asked to leave their audio off unless called upon to speak or they may be asked to comment only in chat. Participants may be asked to leave their video on or to display a photo. Sending an agenda in advance or providing it immediately before the meeting can also help members to prepare, depending on the purpose of the meeting.

**101. D:** The elements of nursing care that are reflected by nursing-sensitive indicators include:

- Structure: Staffing levels/patterns, academic preparation (registered nurse [RN], associate of science [AS], bachelor of science [BS], master of science [MS], and doctor of nursing practice [DNP] degrees), and certifications.
- Process: Patient care procedures, assessment interventions, and job satisfaction.
- Outcomes: Complications (falls, ulcers, heart failure), readmission, length of stay.

**102. C:** If the fiscal year (the budgetary year) at an organization coincides with that of the state legislature and the US Congress, it would run from July 1 to June 30. Many public institutions, such as schools and hospitals, that depend on government support use this fiscal year. Other organizations may use the calendar year, January 1 to December 31, and some use October 1 to September 30.

**103. B:** Meta-analyses and systematic reviews provide the highest level of evidence because they include the results of a number of studies. Systematic reviews summarize literature and findings related to a specific topic, whereas meta-analyses combine data from various research studies. The next highest level of evidence is attained by randomized controlled trials, followed by cohort studies, and then case studies. Expert opinion has the lowest level of evidence and should not be relied on in research because of inherent bias.

**104. D:** After discharge or the last contact with an adult patient, a hospital must keep the patient's health record for varying times, depending on the state. Most states require 5–10 years, but some states have no regulations, and one state (Massachusetts) requires 30 years. Most states require that records for minor patients be kept for a specified number of years after patients reach the age of majority.

**105. C:** Convenience sampling, in which all participants are accepted or participants are chosen in advance, has the highest probability of bias. For quota sampling, participants are chosen according to specific traits, such as participants in different age groups. For purposive sampling, the choice of participants is based on specific criteria. Snowball sampling involves selecting an initial participant who then recommends others.

**106. B:** When developing in-service programs to address deficiencies in care or procedures, the usual place to begin is with the accreditation report because any deficiencies that are noted must be corrected. Other in-service programs may be based on:

- Required content: Mandated courses (state, federal regulations, organizational).
- New developments: Equipment, treatments, best practices.
- Local concerns: Issues such as substance abuse, homelessness.
- National/Future concerns: Dealing with pandemics, changes in demographics.

**107. A:** The most critical aspect of time management is prioritization, determining what needs to be taken care of first and what can be delayed. A tool such as a prioritization matrix may be helpful in establishing priorities. When prioritizing, tasks can usually be categorized:

- Highest priority: Things that are important and urgent.
- High priority: Things that are important but not urgent.
- Moderate priority: Things that are not important but are urgent.
- Low priority: Things that are not important and not urgent.

**108. C:** The first (doing) stage of role transition usually occurs over a period of about 3–4 months.

| Stages of role transition (12 months) | |
|---|---|
| **Doing (3–4 months)** | Transition shock with emotional lability and self-doubt as individuals learn new skills and recognize their limitations. Unsure of responsibilities and expectations. Problem-solving skills are limited. |
| **Being (4–5 months)** | Transition crisis during which knowledge increases along with self-doubt. Continued stress but increased awareness of individual role. May feel unprepared for a clinical position. |
| **Knowing (3–4 months)** | Acceptance of the new role and recovering from some of the problems and stresses of earlier stages, gaining confidence. |

**109. A:** When using Kotter's eight-step change model to integrate findings of evidence-based research into practice, the first phase is to establish urgency. One way to do that is to use statistics to show the extent of a problem, such as the number of hospital readmissions and the resulting loss of income. The next phases are to create a coalition, develop a vision, communicate the vision, empower action, generate short-term wins, consolidate gains/produce momentum, and anchor approaches.

**110. D:** External environment: Threats. SWOT analysis includes:

| Internal environment | | External environment | |
|---|---|---|---|
| Strengths | Weaknesses | Opportunities | Threats |
| Financial stability<br>Programs and services<br>Staff persons<br>Client/Staff satisfaction | Increasing costs<br>Outdated equipment<br>Ineffective programs<br>Marketing | Increased population<br>New programs<br>New markets<br>Stakeholders | Low reimbursement<br>Regulations<br>Competition<br>Political changes |

**111. B:** The four primary core criteria for credentialing and privileging are:

1. Licensure: Must be current through the appropriate state board.
2. Education: Degrees, training, and experience appropriate for the credential.
3. Competence: Evaluations and recommendations by peers regarding clinical competence and judgment provide information about how the person applies knowledge.
4. Performance ability: Demonstrated ability to perform the duties to which the credentialing/privileging applies.

**112. B:** With smart pumps, the most frequent errors are with secondary infusions, which may be delayed because the clamp is not released or may be omitted or administered at the wrong rate or dosage. Other potential errors are associated with dose/rate confusion, mixing up intravenous lines, and entering an incorrect dosage (such as entering a 0 instead of a decimal point or omitting a decimal point). Inclusion of a drug library with alerts can help to reduce errors.

**113. A:** The first step in the educational planning process and assessment is to collect data from multiple sources, including nurses, interdisciplinary teams, consumers, professional organizations, journals, key stakeholders, and regulatory agencies. The NPD practitioner should use current technologies to assess data, use reliable techniques and instruments based on evidence-based techniques, and take note of trends in healthcare. Techniques for data collection may include focus groups, surveys, and literature review.

**114. C:** If the operating budget for the department is reevaluated each budget period to determine if it should be partially or completed funded, it is referred to as a zero-based budget. Other types of budgets include:

- Fixed/Forecast: Revenue and expenses are forecast for the entire budget period, and budget items are fixed.
- Flexible: Estimates are made regarding anticipated changes in revenue and expenses, and fixed and variable costs are identified.
- Continuous/Rolling: Periodic updates to the budget, including revenues, costs, volume, are done prior to the next budget cycle.

**115. D:** During the planning phase when developing strategies for an education program, it is most important for the NPD practitioner to individualize the content to the target learners. The presentation of content, for example, may be quite different if the intended learners represent many different positions and disciplines than if the content is aimed solely at one type of professional. Issues to consider include job responsibilities, educational level, experience, and learning style preferences.

**116. A:** If the NPD practitioner wants to purchase a simulation mannequin for training purposes and the fiscal year starts July 1, the budgetary planning should begin in December, providing 6–7 months of lead time for gathering information about the costs of the equipment and the training costs for use of the equipment. This time period for development of the next annual budget is referred to as the formulation stage, the first stage in budget development, followed by the review and enactment stage and the execution stage.

**117. D:** Internal validity describes the degree to which a researcher can determine that the independent variable produced a change in the dependent variable. External validity is the degree to which the results of the research can be generalized. Construct validity is the degree to which the instrument being used actually measures that which is intended. Statistical conclusion validity is the degree to which the results of statistical analysis reflect the true relationship between dependent and independent variables.

**118. B:** During the implementation stage of an education plan, one of the primary roles of the NPD practitioner is to coordinate various resources and system, including technical, educational, financial, informatics, and administrative, so that the rollout goes smoothly. Another responsibility is to collaborate with learners to ensure that the information shared is evidence-based and that the learning environment is positive, thereby encouraging compliance with the program.

**119. C:** Failure mode and effects analysis is a team-based prospective analysis method that attempts to identify and correct failures in a process before its use to ensure positive outcomes. Steps include:

- Defining: Outline the process in detail.
- Creating a team: Assemble an ad hoc team of those involved in the process or those with expertise.
- Describing: A numbered flowchart describes each step and substep.
- Brainstorming: Each step/substep is analyzed for potential failures.

**120. A:** When using PDSA (also referred to as the Deming cycle) for process improvement, the phase during which the action plan is developed is P (plan). Phases:

- Plan: Opportunities for improvement are identified and prioritized, current processes are described, data are collected, brainstorming takes place, an action plan is developed.
- Do: New processes are tested, and data are collected and analyzed.
- Study: Analysis of the data is completed, and the results are summarized.
- Act: The plan is implemented, problems are identified, data analysis continues.

**121. C:** The most important factor in healthcare customer service is excellence in healthcare; that is, from the first contact to the last, the patient should be shown consideration and respect in all encounters and should be consulted and informed regarding all medications and treatments. Patients tend to remember negative experiences more readily than positive, so patients who feel well cared for are more likely to have a positive reaction to the healthcare organization.

**122. D:** During the evaluation phase of the education design process, it is especially important for learners and other key stakeholders to be engaged in its evaluation. The program should be evaluated in terms of achievement of the anticipated outcomes, which should be clearly outlined for learners. When learners participate in determining the methods of evaluation, they are more likely to view an evaluation as fair and as a necessary component of learning. Evaluation data should always be shared with learners.

**123. B:** The initial strategy in developing a culture of empowerment is to outline expectations so the staff knows what is expected of them and they have the tools to handle their new responsibilities. Empowerment means allowing staff members to make decisions about some aspects of their work; for example, the staff on a unit may be empowered to establish their own work schedules, but they need to be knowledgeable about how schedules work, the staffing models, and budgetary constraints.

**124. A:** For the Skills Base competency management model, the three necessary components are:

1. Ability: Skills and the ability to use and apply knowledge.
2. Desire: Attitude, interests, and motivation.
3. Knowledge: Educational preparation, degrees, certifications, and training.

Competency management is a method of evaluating the ability of the members of an organization to meet the organization's objectives. To demonstrate competence, one must have the proper mix of ability, desire, and knowledge.

**125. D:** Leaving work on time and refusing overtime assignments likely indicate having a healthy work–life balance. Although working overtime hours may be a necessity with a pandemic, it takes a heavy toll on the worker. It is easy to center life around work, but this can negatively impact other aspects of life, such as social and family relationships. Working in a position in which the person feels no reward other than salary can be mentally and physically exhausting, even if the hours are part time.

**126. C:** The purpose of CMS core measures is to produce better patient outcomes for common conditions and to prevent complications. There are adult and pediatric core measures. Adult core measures include controlling high blood pressure, use of high-risk medications in the elderly, preventive care and screening for tobacco use, use of imaging studies for low back pain, preventive care and screening for clinical depression, documentation of current medication in the medical record, preventive care and screening for body mass index, receipt of the specialist report after referral, and functional status assessment for complex chronic conditions. Pediatric core measures include appropriate testing for children with pharyngitis, weight assessment and counseling for nutrition and physical activity, chlamydia screening for women, use of appropriate medications for asthma, immunization status, treatment for upper respiratory infections, follow-up care for children prescribed attention-deficit/hyperactivity disorder medication, preventive care and screening for clinical depression, and care for dental decay or cavities.

**127. B:** If the NPD practitioner asks learners to work together to develop a patient instruction pamphlet as part of a training series, this teaching model is referred to as project based because the learners are tasked with developing materials. Other teaching models include:

- Goal focused: Learners are presented with a goal and all the materials and activities aimed at achieving that goal.
- Problem based: Learners work in teams to solve problems.
- Anchored: Activities are based on problem solving in relation to realistic case studies.

**128. D:** According to the 10-20-30 rule for PowerPoint or other presentation software, the font size for the text should be no smaller than 30 points. The rest of the rule limits the number of slides to no more than 10 and presentations to no more than 20 minutes. It is important when preparing slide presentations for a group to consider the size of the audience, the size of the room, and the size of the projected slides. Slides should be able to be easily read from the back of the room and should contain only the main points of the presentation, not long sentences.

**129. A:** Establishing a culture of safety within an organization requires an initial commitment from leadership, who make clear that safety is the highest priority. Elements that contribute to a culture of safety include encouragement to report errors or mistakes, a supportive rather than punitive approach to mistakes, and ongoing education about the importance of safety and ways in which to improve safety in the environment. A culture of safety means that there is a shared belief among all levels of the organization regarding its importance.

**130. D:** To disseminate research findings to the broadest healthcare audience, the best method is generally publication in a professional journal because those who receive the journal will have access to the research and it will then also show up in database searches on the topic of the research. Publication in the popular press may reach a wider general audience, but not necessarily those in healthcare. Conference presentations are viewed by a limited number of professionals, and journal clubs are usually in house with few members.

**131. C:** An impact evaluation is intended to measure the program's effects on the organization or the greater community. For example, an impact evaluation may help to determine whether a mentoring program for newly hired nurses improves retention over time. One of the primary purposes of an impact evaluation is to determine if a program is cost-effective. Other types of evaluations include process (formative), content, outcome (summative), and program.

**132. B:** The five major functional areas in the hospital emergency incident command system include administrative, logistics, planning, finance, and operations. Disaster/Emergency response plans should be in place for the facility based on the hospital emergency incident command system, which provides a model for management, responsibilities, and communication. The incident commander is part of the administrative area, which also usually includes a public information officer to disseminate information, a liaison officer, and a safety and security officer.

**133. D:** When conducting a root cause analysis, which is a retrospective analysis, it is especially important to identify contributing factors as well as the direct cause. For example, if a patient had a severe reaction to an overdose administered by a nurse who failed to check the dosage, this is the direct cause; however, contributing factors may be understaffing and forced overtime that left the nurse exhausted and distracted. Observations should be objective and not subjective or biased.

**134. C:** When preparing a formal report, a table of contents should be included for documents of more than 10 pages so that readers can easily access the information in the report. Reports should also contain an executive summary that outlines all of the main points. The report itself should contain an introduction, the body of the report, a conclusion, a bibliography/works cited list, and an appendix (if needed).

**135. B:** If an analysis of data shows no outliers, the preferred statistic to report is the mean (the average) because 68% of the data will fall within one standard deviation of the mean. Outliers are those values that lie outside the normal distribution, which may skew the results. Although outliers affect the mean, they have no effect on the mode (the most frequently occurring value) or median (the middle value).

**136. C:** If an employer wants to ask whether a job applicant has a disability that requires accommodation, under the Americans with Disabilities Act, it can be done after the person is hired but before the person starts work; however, the employer must ask all hires in the same job category the same question and cannot single out anyone. If a person has a disability, the law requires that the person disclose it at this point. After the person begins working, the employer can no longer inquire about medical conditions unless the person requests accommodations.

**137. A:** In a just culture, if a nurse who has been caring for a patient for 3 days is observed greeting the patient by name and giving the patient a medication without checking the patient's identification band, an appropriate response would be coaching the nurse and reviewing facility procedures. Errors are classified as:

- Human error: Inadvertent actions, mistakes, or lapses in proper procedure. Management includes consoling the person.
- At-risk behavior: Unjustified risk, choice. Management includes providing incentives for correct behavior and coaching the person.
- Reckless behavior: Conscious disregard for proper procedures. Management includes remedial action and/or punitive action.

**138. D:** The primary purpose of a process evaluation is to make necessary adjustments to the program while it is ongoing. Process evaluations are usually aimed at one class or one lesson. For example, learners may be asked to fill out an evaluation after a class regarding whether the information presented was clear and if enough time was allotted for questions or practice. Based on the responses, alterations may be made in the plans for subsequent classes.

**139. B:** Baby boomers are most likely to enjoy small talk as a way to build relationships and reach consensus and value working as part of a team. Members of the earlier silent generation are much more formal, tend to dislike small talk, and prefer to follow the chain of command. Members of the younger generations, X and Y, are more informal and often see little value in the chain of command and may circumvent their immediate supervisors. Younger generations are also more likely to emphasize the need for a positive work–life balance.

**140. C:** Comparison/Control.

| | | |
|---|---|---|
| **P** | Patient/ Population | List important characteristics (e.g., 35-year-old male with low back pain). |
| **I** | Intervention/ Indicator | Explain the desired intervention under consideration (e.g., acupuncture). |
| **C** | Comparison/ Control | List other possible interventions or alternatives (e.g., surgery). |
| **O** | Outcome | Provide the desired measurable outcomes (e.g., decreased pain levels [from 6–7 to 1–2], and increased mobility). |
| **T** | Time | Time frame (if appropriate) |

**141. B:** The first step in carrying out a needs assessment is to determine the target learners. For example, if the NPD practitioner is planning a program to correct deficiencies identified in an accreditation report, the problem may be organization-wide, restricted to one unit, or applicable to one professional group or even, in some instances, to one individual or to a small group. Developing a program aimed at all staff members may be unnecessary, time-consuming, and costly.

**142. C:** According to TJC, if a sentinel event occurs at a hospital, the hospital must prepare a corrective action plan within 45 business days. Although the hospital is not required to notify TJC when a sentinel event occurs, TJC can provide resources to assist in the hospital's investigation of the event. Sentinel events include those patient safety events that result in death of the patient, permanent harm, or severe life-threatening temporary harm.

**143. D:** Printed materials are the least effective means of providing health information to a population with low health literacy. Low health literacy is often the result of low general literacy or illiteracy, so even preparing materials at a low grade level may not be adequate. Despite this, printed materials are most commonly used to communicate health information. It is important to identify the target population and develop materials suitable for that population.

**144. A:** If using simulations in a lab as part of the orientation of newly hired nurses, the learners should be provided guidelines about specific objectives. During the simulation, the NPD practitioner observes and fills out a checklist of the learner's actions during the simulation without interfering or commenting. At the end of the simulation, a debriefing session should be held with the individual learner or a group of learners during which the learners recount their experience and what they have learned or what they need to work on and the NPD professional provides feedback based on the evaluation checklist and observation.

**145. C:** If a researcher chooses a group of patients without disease, assesses risk factors, and then follows the group over time to determine which ones develop disease, this type of study is a prospective cohort study. For example, this is typical of general surveillance studies for surgical site infections. Cohort studies take more time but are more reliable statistically than case control studies. In another type of cohort study, an exposed group and a nonexposed group may be followed to determine how many develop a particular disease.

**146. A:** If a healthcare organization requires multiple orientation and continuing education courses for a wide range of staff in four different locations, the best management method is likely to use an LMS, such as Relias or HealthStream Learning, specifically designed for healthcare. LMSs are used to create, deliver, track, grade, and report on coursework and can provide all of the necessary materials online. An LMS can be used in lieu of or in support of face-to-face instruction.

**147. D:** When developing a Gantt chart to set a timeline for program management, start-to-finish dependencies require that the predecessor begins before the successor ends. Dependencies refer to the relationship between different tasks with the predecessor occurring first. Other dependency relationships include finish-to-finish, in which the predecessor ends before the successor ends. With start-to-start dependency, the predecessor must begin before the successor. Finish-to-start dependency requires that the predecessor ends before the successor begins.

**148. B:** If, during a brainstorming session about quality improvement processes, the participants begin judging suggestions as they are contributed, the role of the NPD practitioner is to bring participants back to only expressing ideas first, by saying, for example, "Let's finish making a list of ideas first, and then we'll go through them one at a time and discuss the pros and cons." Judgments presented during the initial brainstorming can impede the flow of ideas and may make some participants feel intimidated.

**149. D:** When carrying out evidence-based research and testing the reliability of instruments, the three important attributes include:

1. Stability: Repeated testing under the same circumstances renders the same scores.
2. Equivalence: Alternate raters or forms of an instrument are in agreement and achieve the same results.
3. Internal consistency (aka homogeneity): All items present in an instrument measure the same concept.

**150. C:** Expenditures for advertising to promote a healthcare program are referred to as sunk costs because the money is spent and cannot be recovered. Sunk costs are common in organizations and can, for example, include the cost of leasing a building. Variable costs can increase or decrease based on volume, such as food costs that vary according to patient census. Operating costs are those that are necessary for running the organization as a business, such as office staff and supplies.

# How to Overcome Test Anxiety

Just the thought of taking a test is enough to make most people a little nervous. A test is an important event that can have a long-term impact on your future, so it's important to take it seriously and it's natural to feel anxious about performing well. But just because anxiety is normal, that doesn't mean that it's helpful in test taking, or that you should simply accept it as part of your life. Anxiety can have a variety of effects. These effects can be mild, like making you feel slightly nervous, or severe, like blocking your ability to focus or remember even a simple detail.

If you experience test anxiety—whether severe or mild—it's important to know how to beat it. To discover this, first you need to understand what causes test anxiety.

## Causes of Test Anxiety

While we often think of anxiety as an uncontrollable emotional state, it can actually be caused by simple, practical things. One of the most common causes of test anxiety is that a person does not feel adequately prepared for their test. This feeling can be the result of many different issues such as poor study habits or lack of organization, but the most common culprit is time management. Starting to study too late, failing to organize your study time to cover all of the material, or being distracted while you study will mean that you're not well prepared for the test. This may lead to cramming the night before, which will cause you to be physically and mentally exhausted for the test. Poor time management also contributes to feelings of stress, fear, and hopelessness as you realize you are not well prepared but don't know what to do about it.

Other times, test anxiety is not related to your preparation for the test but comes from unresolved fear. This may be a past failure on a test, or poor performance on tests in general. It may come from comparing yourself to others who seem to be performing better or from the stress of living up to expectations. Anxiety may be driven by fears of the future—how failure on this test would affect your educational and career goals. These fears are often completely irrational, but they can still negatively impact your test performance.

**Review Video: 3 Reasons You Have Test Anxiety**
Visit mometrix.com/academy and enter code: 428468

## Elements of Test Anxiety

As mentioned earlier, test anxiety is considered to be an emotional state, but it has physical and mental components as well. Sometimes you may not even realize that you are suffering from test anxiety until you notice the physical symptoms. These can include trembling hands, rapid heartbeat, sweating, nausea, and tense muscles. Extreme anxiety may lead to fainting or vomiting. Obviously, any of these symptoms can have a negative impact on testing. It is important to recognize them as soon as they begin to occur so that you can address the problem before it damages your performance.

**Review Video: 3 Ways to Tell You Have Test Anxiety**
Visit mometrix.com/academy and enter code: 927847

The mental components of test anxiety include trouble focusing and inability to remember learned information. During a test, your mind is on high alert, which can help you recall information and stay focused for an extended period of time. However, anxiety interferes with your mind's natural processes, causing you to blank out, even on the questions you know well. The strain of testing during anxiety makes it difficult to stay focused, especially on a test that may take several hours. Extreme anxiety can take a huge mental toll, making it difficult not only to recall test information but even to understand the test questions or pull your thoughts together.

**Review Video: How Test Anxiety Affects Memory**
Visit mometrix.com/academy and enter code: 609003

## Effects of Test Anxiety

Test anxiety is like a disease—if left untreated, it will get progressively worse. Anxiety leads to poor performance, and this reinforces the feelings of fear and failure, which in turn lead to poor performances on subsequent tests. It can grow from a mild nervousness to a crippling condition. If allowed to progress, test anxiety can have a big impact on your schooling, and consequently on your future.

Test anxiety can spread to other parts of your life. Anxiety on tests can become anxiety in any stressful situation, and blanking on a test can turn into panicking in a job situation. But fortunately, you don't have to let anxiety rule your testing and determine your grades. There are a number of relatively simple steps you can take to move past anxiety and function normally on a test and in the rest of life.

**Review Video: How Test Anxiety Impacts Your Grades**
Visit mometrix.com/academy and enter code: 939819

## Physical Steps for Beating Test Anxiety

While test anxiety is a serious problem, the good news is that it can be overcome. It doesn't have to control your ability to think and remember information. While it may take time, you can begin taking steps today to beat anxiety.

Just as your first hint that you may be struggling with anxiety comes from the physical symptoms, the first step to treating it is also physical. Rest is crucial for having a clear, strong mind. If you are tired, it is much easier to give in to anxiety. But if you establish good sleep habits, your body and mind will be ready to perform optimally, without the strain of exhaustion. Additionally, sleeping well helps you to retain information better, so you're more likely to recall the answers when you see the test questions.

Getting good sleep means more than going to bed on time. It's important to allow your brain time to relax. Take study breaks from time to time so it doesn't get overworked, and don't study right before bed. Take time to rest your mind before trying to rest your body, or you may find it difficult to fall asleep.

**Review Video: The Importance of Sleep for Your Brain**
Visit mometrix.com/academy and enter code: 319338

Along with sleep, other aspects of physical health are important in preparing for a test. Good nutrition is vital for good brain function. Sugary foods and drinks may give a burst of energy but this burst is followed by a crash, both physically and emotionally. Instead, fuel your body with protein and vitamin-rich foods.

Also, drink plenty of water. Dehydration can lead to headaches and exhaustion, especially if your brain is already under stress from the rigors of the test. Particularly if your test is a long one, drink water during the breaks. And if possible, take an energy-boosting snack to eat between sections.

**Review Video: How Diet Can Affect your Mood**
Visit mometrix.com/academy and enter code: 624317

Along with sleep and diet, a third important part of physical health is exercise. Maintaining a steady workout schedule is helpful, but even taking 5-minute study breaks to walk can help get your blood pumping faster and clear your head. Exercise also releases endorphins, which contribute to a positive feeling and can help combat test anxiety.

When you nurture your physical health, you are also contributing to your mental health. If your body is healthy, your mind is much more likely to be healthy as well. So take time to rest, nourish your body with healthy food and water, and get moving as much as possible. Taking these physical steps will make you stronger and more able to take the mental steps necessary to overcome test anxiety.

## Mental Steps for Beating Test Anxiety

Working on the mental side of test anxiety can be more challenging, but as with the physical side, there are clear steps you can take to overcome it. As mentioned earlier, test anxiety often stems from lack of preparation, so the obvious solution is to prepare for the test. Effective studying may be the most important weapon you have for beating test anxiety, but you can and should employ several other mental tools to combat fear.

First, boost your confidence by reminding yourself of past success—tests or projects that you aced. If you're putting as much effort into preparing for this test as you did for those, there's no reason you should expect to fail here. Work hard to prepare; then trust your preparation.

Second, surround yourself with encouraging people. It can be helpful to find a study group, but be sure that the people you're around will encourage a positive attitude. If you spend time with others who are anxious or cynical, this will only contribute to your own anxiety. Look for others who are motivated to study hard from a desire to succeed, not from a fear of failure.

Third, reward yourself. A test is physically and mentally tiring, even without anxiety, and it can be helpful to have something to look forward to. Plan an activity following the test, regardless of the outcome, such as going to a movie or getting ice cream.

When you are taking the test, if you find yourself beginning to feel anxious, remind yourself that you know the material. Visualize successfully completing the test. Then take a few deep, relaxing breaths and return to it. Work through the questions carefully but with confidence, knowing that you are capable of succeeding.

Developing a healthy mental approach to test taking will also aid in other areas of life. Test anxiety affects more than just the actual test—it can be damaging to your mental health and even contribute to depression. It's important to beat test anxiety before it becomes a problem for more than testing.

**Review Video: Test Anxiety and Depression**
Visit mometrix.com/academy and enter code: 904704

# Study Strategy

Being prepared for the test is necessary to combat anxiety, but what does being prepared look like? You may study for hours on end and still not feel prepared. What you need is a strategy for test prep. The next few pages outline our recommended steps to help you plan out and conquer the challenge of preparation.

## Step 1: Scope Out the Test

Learn everything you can about the format (multiple choice, essay, etc.) and what will be on the test. Gather any study materials, course outlines, or sample exams that may be available. Not only will this help you to prepare, but knowing what to expect can help to alleviate test anxiety.

## Step 2: Map Out the Material

Look through the textbook or study guide and make note of how many chapters or sections it has. Then divide these over the time you have. For example, if a book has 15 chapters and you have five days to study, you need to cover three chapters each day. Even better, if you have the time, leave an extra day at the end for overall review after you have gone through the material in depth.

If time is limited, you may need to prioritize the material. Look through it and make note of which sections you think you already have a good grasp on, and which need review. While you are studying, skim quickly through the familiar sections and take more time on the challenging parts. Write out your plan so you don't get lost as you go. Having a written plan also helps you feel more in control of the study, so anxiety is less likely to arise from feeling overwhelmed at the amount to cover.

## Step 3: Gather Your Tools

Decide what study method works best for you. Do you prefer to highlight in the book as you study and then go back over the highlighted portions? Or do you type out notes of the important information? Or is it helpful to make flashcards that you can carry with you? Assemble the pens, index cards, highlighters, post-it notes, and any other materials you may need so you won't be distracted by getting up to find things while you study.

If you're having a hard time retaining the information or organizing your notes, experiment with different methods. For example, try color-coding by subject with colored pens, highlighters, or post-it notes. If you learn better by hearing, try recording yourself reading your notes so you can listen while in the car, working out, or simply sitting at your desk. Ask a friend to quiz you from your flashcards, or try teaching someone the material to solidify it in your mind.

## Step 4: Create Your Environment

It's important to avoid distractions while you study. This includes both the obvious distractions like visitors and the subtle distractions like an uncomfortable chair (or a too-comfortable couch that makes you want to fall asleep). Set up the best study environment possible: good lighting and a comfortable work area. If background music helps you focus, you may want to turn it on, but otherwise keep the room quiet. If you are using a computer to take notes, be sure you don't have any other windows open, especially applications like social media, games, or anything else that could distract you. Silence your phone and turn off notifications. Be sure to keep water close by so you stay hydrated while you study (but avoid unhealthy drinks and snacks).

Also, take into account the best time of day to study. Are you freshest first thing in the morning? Try to set aside some time then to work through the material. Is your mind clearer in the afternoon or evening? Schedule your study session then. Another method is to study at the same time of day that you will take the test, so that your brain gets used to working on the material at that time and will be ready to focus at test time.

## Step 5: Study!

Once you have done all the study preparation, it's time to settle into the actual studying. Sit down, take a few moments to settle your mind so you can focus, and begin to follow your study plan. Don't give in to distractions or let yourself procrastinate. This is your time to prepare so you'll be ready to fearlessly approach the test. Make the most of the time and stay focused.

Of course, you don't want to burn out. If you study too long you may find that you're not retaining the information very well. Take regular study breaks. For example, taking five minutes out of every hour to walk briskly, breathing deeply and swinging your arms, can help your mind stay fresh.

As you get to the end of each chapter or section, it's a good idea to do a quick review. Remind yourself of what you learned and work on any difficult parts. When you feel that you've mastered the material, move on to the next part. At the end of your study session, briefly skim through your notes again.

But while review is helpful, cramming last minute is NOT. If at all possible, work ahead so that you won't need to fit all your study into the last day. Cramming overloads your brain with more information than it can process and retain, and your tired mind may struggle to recall even previously learned information when it is overwhelmed with last-minute study. Also, the urgent nature of cramming and the stress placed on your brain contribute to anxiety. You'll be more likely to go to the test feeling unprepared and having trouble thinking clearly.

So don't cram, and don't stay up late before the test, even just to review your notes at a leisurely pace. Your brain needs rest more than it needs to go over the information again. In fact, plan to finish your studies by noon or early afternoon the day before the test. Give your brain the rest of the day to relax or focus on other things, and get a good night's sleep. Then you will be fresh for the test and better able to recall what you've studied.

## Step 6: Take a practice test

Many courses offer sample tests, either online or in the study materials. This is an excellent resource to check whether you have mastered the material, as well as to prepare for the test format and environment.

Check the test format ahead of time: the number of questions, the type (multiple choice, free response, etc.), and the time limit. Then create a plan for working through them. For example, if you have 30 minutes to take a 60-question test, your limit is 30 seconds per question. Spend less time on the questions you know well so that you can take more time on the difficult ones.

If you have time to take several practice tests, take the first one open book, with no time limit. Work through the questions at your own pace and make sure you fully understand them. Gradually work up to taking a test under test conditions: sit at a desk with all study materials put away and set a timer. Pace yourself to make sure you finish the test with time to spare and go back to check your answers if you have time.

After each test, check your answers. On the questions you missed, be sure you understand why you missed them. Did you misread the question (tests can use tricky wording)? Did you forget the information? Or was it something you hadn't learned? Go back and study any shaky areas that the practice tests reveal.

Taking these tests not only helps with your grade, but also aids in combating test anxiety. If you're already used to the test conditions, you're less likely to worry about it, and working through tests until you're scoring well gives you a confidence boost. Go through the practice tests until you feel comfortable, and then you can go into the test knowing that you're ready for it.

## Test Tips

On test day, you should be confident, knowing that you've prepared well and are ready to answer the questions. But aside from preparation, there are several test day strategies you can employ to maximize your performance.

First, as stated before, get a good night's sleep the night before the test (and for several nights before that, if possible). Go into the test with a fresh, alert mind rather than staying up late to study.

Try not to change too much about your normal routine on the day of the test. It's important to eat a nutritious breakfast, but if you normally don't eat breakfast at all, consider eating just a protein bar. If you're a coffee drinker, go ahead and have your normal coffee. Just make sure you time it so that the caffeine doesn't wear off right in the middle of your test. Avoid sugary beverages, and drink enough water to stay hydrated but not so much that you need a restroom break 10 minutes into the test. If your test isn't first thing in the morning, consider going for a walk or doing a light workout before the test to get your blood flowing.

Allow yourself enough time to get ready, and leave for the test with plenty of time to spare so you won't have the anxiety of scrambling to arrive in time. Another reason to be early is to select a good seat. It's helpful to sit away from doors and windows, which can be distracting. Find a good seat, get out your supplies, and settle your mind before the test begins.

When the test begins, start by going over the instructions carefully, even if you already know what to expect. Make sure you avoid any careless mistakes by following the directions.

Then begin working through the questions, pacing yourself as you've practiced. If you're not sure on an answer, don't spend too much time on it, and don't let it shake your confidence. Either skip it and come back later, or eliminate as many wrong answers as possible and guess among the remaining ones. Don't dwell on these questions as you continue—put them out of your mind and focus on what lies ahead.

Be sure to read all of the answer choices, even if you're sure the first one is the right answer. Sometimes you'll find a better one if you keep reading. But don't second-guess yourself if you do immediately know the answer. Your gut instinct is usually right. Don't let test anxiety rob you of the information you know.

If you have time at the end of the test (and if the test format allows), go back and review your answers. Be cautious about changing any, since your first instinct tends to be correct, but make sure you didn't misread any of the questions or accidentally mark the wrong answer choice. Look over any you skipped and make an educated guess.

At the end, leave the test feeling confident. You've done your best, so don't waste time worrying about your performance or wishing you could change anything. Instead, celebrate the successful completion of this test. And finally, use this test to learn how to deal with anxiety even better next time.

**Review Video: 5 Tips to Beat Test Anxiety**
Visit mometrix.com/academy and enter code: 570656

## Important Qualification

Not all anxiety is created equal. If your test anxiety is causing major issues in your life beyond the classroom or testing center, or if you are experiencing troubling physical symptoms related to your anxiety, it may be a sign of a serious physiological or psychological condition. If this sounds like your situation, we strongly encourage you to seek professional help.

# Thank You

We at Mometrix would like to extend our heartfelt thanks to you, our friend and patron, for allowing us to play a part in your journey. It is a privilege to serve people from all walks of life who are unified in their commitment to building the best future they can for themselves.

The preparation you devote to these important testing milestones may be the most valuable educational opportunity you have for making a real difference in your life. We encourage you to put your heart into it—that feeling of succeeding, overcoming, and yes, conquering will be well worth the hours you've invested.

We want to hear your story, your struggles and your successes, and if you see any opportunities for us to improve our materials so we can help others even more effectively in the future, please share that with us as well. **The team at Mometrix would be absolutely thrilled to hear from you!** So please, send us an email (support@mometrix.com) and let's stay in touch.

**If you'd like some additional help, check out these other resources we offer for your exam:**
**http://MometrixFlashcards.com/NursingProfDev**

# Additional Bonus Material

Due to our efforts to try to keep this book to a manageable length, we've created a link that will give you access to all of your additional bonus material:

**mometrix.com/bonus948/nursingprofdev**